EENT eye, ear, nose, throat
EHT essential hypertension
EIA enzyme immunoassay
EKG electrocardiogram
ELISA enzyme-linked immunosorbent assay
EMG electromyography
EMS emergency medical services
emul emulsion
endo endometrium
ENT ear, nose, throat
ER emergency room
ESR erythrocyte sedimentation rate
est established; estimated
et and
etiol etiology
Ex examination
exam examination
exc excision
expl lap exploratory laparoscopy
ext external; extract

F

F Fahrenheit
FACP Fellow of the American College of Physicians
FACS Fellow of the American College of Surgeons
FB foreign body
FBS fasting blood sugar
FDLMP first day last menstrual period
Fe iron
FH family history
FHS fetal heart sound
fl fluid
fl dr fluid dram
fl oz fluid ounce
fluor fluoroscopy
ft feet; foot
F/U follow-up
FU follow-up
FUO fever of undetermined origin
Fx fracture
FYI for your information

G

g gram
G gauge
GA gastric analysis
gb gallbladder
GB gallbladder
GC gonorrhea culture

GGE generalized glandular enlargement
GI gastrointestinal
gm gram
gr grain
grav how many pregnancies (*gravida*)
GSW gun-shot wound
gt drop
gtt drops
GTT glucose tolerance test
GU genitourinary
Gyn gynecology
GYN gynecology

H

h hour
H hospital call; hospital consultation; hour
HA headache
Hb hemoglobin
HBP high blood pressure
HC hospital call; hospital consultation; head circumference
HCD house call day
HCL hydrochloric acid
HCN house call night
Hct hematocrit
HCT hematocrit
HCVD hypertensive cardiovascular disease
HEENT head, eyes, ears, nose, throat
hgb hemoglobin
H&H hematocrit and hemoglobin
hist history
HIV human immunodeficiency virus
H_2O water
H_2O_2 hydrogen peroxide
hosp hospital
H&P history and physical (exam)
HPF high-power field
HPI history of present illness
HPIP history, physical (exam), impression, plan
hrs hours
hs bedtime; hour of sleep
HS hospital surgery
HT height
htn hypertension
HV hospital visit
Hx history

Hx/Px history and physical examination
hypo hypodermic

I

IC initial consultation
ICU intensive care unit
I&D incision and drainage
ID intradermal
i.e. that is
IM intramuscular
imp impression
inf infected
inflam inflammation
init initial
inj injection
ins insurance
int internal
I&O intake and output
IPPB intermittent positive pressure breathing
IQ intelligence quotient
ISG immune serum globulin
IT inhalation therapy
IUD intrauterine device
IV intravenous
IVP intravenous pyelogram

K

K potassium
kg kilogram
KOH potassium hyrdroxide
KUB kidneys, ureters, bladder

L

L laboratory; left; liter
L&A light and accommodation
Lab laboratory
LAB laboratory
lac laceration
lat lateral
LBP low blood pressure; low back pain
lb(s) pound(s)
LC large blood pressure cuff
liq liquid
LLQ left lower quadrant
LMP last menstrual period
LPF low-power field
LPF low pressure fluid
LRQ lower right quadrant
LSS lumbosacral spine
lt left
ltd limited
LUQ left upper quadrant
L&W living and well

continued on inside back cover

Delmar's Clinical Handbook
for
Health Care Professionals

Michelle Heller, CMA, RMA

Connie Krebs, CMA-C, BGS

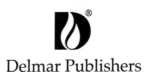

Delmar Publishers

an International Thomson Publishing company I(T)P®

Albany • Bonn • Boston • Cincinnati • Detroit • London • Madrid
Melbourne • Mexico City • New York • Pacific Grove • Paris • San Francisco
Singapore • Tokyo • Toronto • Washington

NOTICE TO THE READER

Cover Design: joanne beckmann design

Visual Identification Guide: courtesy of Medical Economics

Delmar Staff
Publisher: Susan Simpfenderfer
Acquisitions Editor: Marion Waldman
Developmental Editor: Helen V. Yackel
Project Development Editor: Melissa Conan
Production Coordinator: Cathleen Berry
Art and Design Coordinator: Richard Killar
Editorial Assistant: Sarah Holle
Marketing Manager: Darryl Caron

Online Services

Delmar Online
To access a wide variety of Delmar products and services on the World Wide Web, point your browser to:
http://www.delmar.com/delmar.html
or email: info@delmar.com

thomson.com
To access International Thomson Publishing's home site for information on more than 34 publishers and 20,000 products, point your browser to:
http://www.thomson.com
or email: findit@kiosk.thomson.com

COPYRIGHT © 1997
By Delmar Publishers

A division of International Thomson Publishing Inc.

The ITP logo is a trademark under license.

Printed in the United States of America

For more information, contact:

Delmar Publishers
3 Columbia Circle, Box 15015
Albany, New York 12212-5015

International Thomson Publishing Europe
Berkshire House 168-173
High Holborn
London, WC1V 7AA
England

Thomas Nelson Australia
102 Dodds Street
South Melbourne, 3205
Victoria, Australia

Nelson Canada
1120 Birchmount Road
Scarborough, Ontario
Canada, M1K 5G4

International Thomson Editores
Campos Eliseos 385, Piso 7
Col Polanco
11560 Mexico D F Mexico

International Thomson Publishing GmbH
Konigswinterer Strasse 418
53227 Bonn
Germany

International Thomson Publishing Asia
221 Henderson Road
#05-10 Henderson Building
Singapore 0315

International Thomson Publishing Japan
Hirakawacho Kyowa Building, 3F
2-2-1 Hirakawacho
Chiyoda-ku, Tokyo 102
Japan

    3 4 5 6 7 8 9 10 XXX 02 01 00 99 98 97

Library of Congress Cataloging-in-Publication Data
RC55.H45 1997
  Delmar's clinical handbook for health care professionals/
  Michelle Heller, Connie Krebs
    p. cm.
  Includes bibliographical references.
  ISBN 0–8273–7789–4
  1. Internal medicine—Handbooks, manuals, etc. I Krebs, Connie.
  II. Title.
  [DNLM: 1. Clinical Medicine—handbooks. WB 39 H477d 1997]
  616 --dc20
  DNLM/DLC
for Library of Congress   96–20597
                                                  CIP

I would like to dedicate this book to my grandmother, Delma C. Miller, who passed away while this book was being written. To the woman who taught me that hard work and discipline, wrapped in love, reaps many rewards, thank-you Grandma!

Michelle Heller, CMA, RMA

This book is also dedicated to all professionals in the health care field as they administer daily to the needs of the sick, often with little thanks—you are appreciated.

Connie Krebs, CMA-C, BGS

Finding Information in This Book

By matching the numbered guides at the edge of the opposite page with their corresponding tabs along the edge of the book, you can quickly turn to the section containing the material you want.

Contents

SECTION 9   **PROCEDURES, TIPS, AND FACTS**

Preface

The purpose of this handbook is to provide a quick and easy reference to people who plan to work, or are currently working, in family practice, pediatrics, and obstetrics and gynecology offices. Information is provided to the user in an easy, concise, simplistic reference chart format. The charts are comprehensive in content and aid in the complex tasks of patient triage and/or assessment. Charting tips about procedures, troubleshooting, instruments, and tray setups are among the many areas of information to help the medical care provider perform duties for the patient with accuracy and confidence. This handbook also may prove beneficial to the student who is preparing for a career in the field of medical assisting.

This handbook has been written with an emphasis on the complexities of assisting with managed care. This is vitally important because a large portion of offices have accepted some form of managed care.

Listed below are ways in which this handbook can be helpful:

1. Medical assisting students: This handbook will be useful for students to take into the medical laboratory. The handbook's size gives students more room to work than with the bulkier textbooks. The medical assessment charts not only inform students how to assess, but also help them anticipate what the physician will need prior to, during, or following an exam. The medical documentation charts will help students become proficient at charting before they enter the field. Procedure charts will help with recall when a student forgets something, as well as provide tips that will ensure the success of the procedure. (This book is not meant to replace quality instruction or take the place of a textbook, but to complement or serve as a reference in addition to class instruction.)

2. New graduates: This handbook will be particularly beneficial to new graduates. It will help fill in the gaps where needed and will give new graduates that extra boost of confidence.

3. Established assistants: This handbook will help provide the necessary information when assistants forget a small detail or step. It also will help those who have been working in a specialty and now find themselves working in a more complex setting with many more responsibilities.

4. Office supervisors: This handbook will help promote consistency from one employee to the next. It also can be useful in those offices that do not have an office procedure manual in place.

This handbook has been designed so that each section can be personalized according to the individual practices of the office. Most of the charts contain extra lines or space to add information. Several blank charts are included in Section 12. You also will find a place for the physician to sign off on each assessment and documentation chart. This will help ensure consistency between the office staff and the physician. It also will help to cut down on potential legal problems that can occur later.

The inside front and back covers of this book contain common abbreviations that are used in many medical establishments. The pharmacology section provides the user with charts that list medications commonly prescribed today, along with their generic names, classifications, and schedules. A color insert of the most commonly prescribed drugs also is included.

The contents of this book are not standards but suggestions that may make life a little easier in the medical office. ***In many offices, the physician will be the only one who will have the authority to diagnose and prescribe, however, physician assistants and nurse practitioners also have a role in diagnosing and prescribing. Know the chain of command for the establishment with which you are associated.***

It is our hope that by using this reference book, it will make your job much easier.

Acknowledgments

A big thank-you is extended to my family, who supported me throughout this project. To Erin, Megan, and Kevin, thanks for excusing me from many of my motherly duties. To my husband Kevin, who assumed the duties of mom and dad and kept the late-night snacks coming in, thank-you, I love you all! Many thanks to my mother and father, Walter and Judith Allen, who gave me lots of encouragement during this project and helped me with the drug section. I certainly don't want to forget my brother and sister-in-law, Tim and Linda Heller, who had to rescue me from one computer mess after another. To Dan and Theresa Heller, who provided baby-sitting and many meals, thank-you! A big thank-you to all the staff, faculty, and students at Columbus Para-Professional Institute (Columbus, Ohio, Branch), who provided me with much support while completing this project. Many, many thanks to my co-author Connie Krebs for taking on this project when she had many other things going on. Thanks to Helen Yackel and Melissa Conan, my editors at Delmar for their support. And a special thanks to all of my other family members and friends, who supported me with their time, love, and prayers.

Michelle Heller, CMA, RMA

My heartfelt appreciation is extended to Michelle Heller, CMA, for asking me to be a part of this much-needed book for those in the health care field. It was Michelle who had the vision and goal of putting this reference handbook together and I am honored to be a part of seeing this project to fruition. Her dedication and passion in reaching this goal are truly admirable.

My thanks to Helen Yackel, Developmental Editor, for believing in our goal and helping us reach it. And to Melissa Conan, Project Development Editor, for all her assistance in completing this handbook.

Sincere gratitude also is extended to all those people who contributed in various ways in providing us with current information, expertise, suggestions, advice, support, and encouragement.

Connie Krebs, CMA-C, BGS

The authors and the project team at Delmar Publishers also wish to express their appreciation to a dedicated group of professionals who reviewed and provided commentary on the manuscript at various stages.

Jennifer Barr, MEd, CMA, Sinclair Community College, Dayton, OH; Keith A. Blakely, M.D. (Family Practice); Ginny Forrester, R.N., St. Ann's Hospital, Columbus, OH; David Henderson, M.D. (Pediatrician), Cigna Health Care, Columbus, OH; Marsha Holtsberry, CMA, RMA/AMT, EMT-A, Instructor Medical Assisting Program, Columbus Para-Professional Institute; Vickie Johnson, CMA, Tri-County Family Physicians, Canal Winchester, OH; Linda Sue Johnson, CMA, Lenoir Community College, Kinston, NC; Doug Katula, M.D., (Internal Medicine), Central Ohio Prime Care; John P. Keefe, RPA-C, Executive Park East, Albany, NY; Deborah J. Kennedy, M.D. (OB-GYN), Women Physicians in OB-GYN; Joan E. King, D.O. (Internal Medicine), Northwest Internal Medicine, Columbus, OH; Eric Legg, M.D. (Family Practice), Tri-County Family Physicians, Canal Winchester, OH; Fran Muller, MEd, Gilford Technical Community College, Jamestown, NC; John Nance, RMA, Medical Assisting Instructor, Columbus Para-Professional Institute; Helen Neff, CMA, Tri-County Family Physicians, Canal Winchester, OH; Imagene O'Bryan, RMA, Central Ohio Prime Care, Columbus, OH; Wanda Orsett, LPN, CMA, Wake Technical Community College, Raleigh, NC; Tom George Peponis, Jr, D.O. (Family Practice), Columbus, OH; Theresa Perry, MS, CMA, Husson College, Bangor, ME; Jean Riddell, MA, CMA, Suffolk Community College, Medical Assisting Program, Selden, NY; Linda Scarborough, RN, Lanier Technical Institute, Oakwood, GA; Heather Smith, RMA, Columbus OB-GYN, Columbus, OH; Lois Smith, RN, Arapahoe Community College, Littleton, CO; Lee A. Speck, MT (AMT), MLT (ASCP), Corning Metpath Laboratories, Columbus, OH; Kimberly Stischok, RMA, Dr. Tom Peponis, Columbus, OH; Elesa Stout, R.T., R, Children's Hospital Radiology Department, Columbus, OH; Fauna Stout, B.S., Health Education, CMA, RMA/AMT, Northwest Internal Medicine, Columbus, OH; Diane Tallo, M.D. (Endocrinologist), Central Ohio Prime Care, Columbus, OH; Warner M. Thomas, Jr., Atty, McCarthy & Palmer Law Firm, Columbus, OH; Donna Waites R.Ph, Mt. Carmel East Hospital, Columbus, OH.

SECTION

1

MANAGED CARE

Introduction

U ntil a few years ago, the handling of insurance in the medical office was largely an administrative function. In today's medical office, it is everyone's responsibility.

Insurance companies govern much of what is done for patients. As a clinical assistant in a medical establishment, you must constantly update yourself with each insurance company's policies and procedures.

Insurance protocol may have a direct bearing on managing patient care in the following situations:

1. Authorizing a patient to go to the emergency room: Many managed care plans require authorization from a primary care physician before going to an emergency room, unless it is a life-threatening condition.

2. Referring a patient to a specialist: Many insurance companies require that a patient see their primary care physician before consulting a specialist.

3. Performing various laboratory tests on a patient: Many insurance companies require that certain laboratory tests be performed at specific facilities or be sent to specific reference labs.

4. Pre-Certification: Many insurance companies require pre-certification for various diagnostic and medical procedures and hospitalizations. This means that authorization must be obtained, either by telephone or in writing, from the insurance company prior to the procedure being performed. Failure to do so might result in nonpayment for the procedure.

5. Participating provider: Some procedures do not have to be precertified but require that a patient be sent to a specific facility for the procedure. Failure to do so might result in nonpayment by the insurance company.

Always double check a patient's insurance coverage before considering any of the above situations.

Section 12 of this book contains a sample pre-certification form.

To save the assistant time, most insurance companies allow forms to be faxed rather than waiting for telephone authorization.

Insurance companies usually provide caregivers with manuals that explain the proper policies and procedures to be followed. Phone numbers, referral lists, and other pertinent information also are provided.

Section 12 of this book contains a blank form than can be photocopied and used for quick reference when manuals cannot be easily obtained. This form provides the user with information such as phone numbers, pre-certification requirements, and participating provider information for each plan for which the caregiver has a contract.

Insurance procedures and policies are rapidly changing. The smart assistant will continually strive to keep abreast of the latest changes in each plan.

Medical Records Management Checklist

The following is a sample of what types of information an insurance reviewer might look for when doing a chart review, which highlights the records management portion of an inspection. Keep in mind that these are general guidelines and in no way reflect each component observed by each insurance company. Although some insurance companies will provide an office with a checklist before its visit, others may not.

1. SECURITY OF RECORDS

   A. What is being done to ensure that records are secure and safe from physical harm?

   B. What is being done to make sure that records remain confidential?

   C. How are active records separated from inactive records?

   D. Is there a list of initials and signatures of all personnel who make chart entries?

   E. How long are records retained? (Do they meet the guidelines of the plan?)

   F. Are records kept in some type of a jacket, labeled with a patient's name?

   G. Do the charts reflect, both on the inside and outside, what type of insurance a patient has?

   H. Does each page in the chart reflect a patient's identity?

   I. Does the office have a tracking log that follows up on patients who break appointments?

   J. Are patients' drug allergies flagged on the outside of the chart as well as on the inside?

   K. Can records be easily retrieved?

2. PREVENTATIVE MEDICINE MEASURES

   A. Are established patients offered an annual exam? (This would vary, depending on the patient's individual plan.)

B. What type of follow-up procedures does the office employ to notify female patients of their annual pap exams or mammograms?

C. Are pediatric schedules provided for custodial guardians so they know when to schedule their child's immunizations?

D. Does your office have a plan to track patients who fall behind on their immunizations?

3. MEDICAL RECORD CONTENTS

A. Are medical records organized and easy to follow?

B. Does your office have a complete database for each established patient that contains:

- a complete personal medical history

- a complete familial medical history

- a complete social history, reflecting smoking, recreational drug, and alcohol habits, as well as exercise, hobbies, etc.

- a complete menstrual and pregnancy history on each female patient

C. Does each chief complaint and progress note reflect the following information:

- subjective findings

- objective findings

- diagnosis

- treatment/follow-up care

- patient education

D. Are all entries dated?

E. Are all entries in chronological order?

F. Are all entries properly signed or initialed by appropriate personnel?

G. Has the physician initialed all entries made by himself or herself, as well as other staff members? (This will vary from one insurance company to another.)

H. Are weights, heights, and blood pressures being documented as often as the insurance company mandates?

I. Are charts arranged so chronic medical problems can be easily identified?

J. Is each section of the chart separate from one another for easy access, i.e., progress notes, diagnostic findings, correspondences, and so on?

K. Does the chart have an immunization log and a current medication log that can be easily retrieved in an emergency situation (i.e., on the cover, front, or rear of the chart)?

L. Do all medications administered in the office contain the following information?

- name of the medication
- dose or strength of the medication
- route of administration
- site of administration
- time of administration (when it applies)
- who ordered the medication
- who administered the medication

In the case of immunizations, is the following information listed?

- manufacturer's name
- lot #
- expiration date

M. Are all samples that are given to patients properly documented?

N. Are orders for each diagnostic procedure properly documented?

O. Does your office have orders from consulting physicians, i.e., for blood work or Xrays that are to be performed at your facility, written on a prescription blank or another type of form? (Many insurance companies will not accept a telephone order.)

P. Does all prescription documentation contain the following?

- date
- name of pharmacy (including location and telephone number)
- full name of pharmacist
- name of drug
- strength of drug

- amount dispensed (when it applies)
- patient instructions
- number of refills
- who ordered the prescription
- who called it in

Q. Are copies of consultations filed in the charts?

R. Are in-patient procedures documented?

S. Are all broken appointments as well as rescheduled appointments documented in the chart?

T. Is there a completed growth chart on every patient eighteen years old and under?

U. Are all entries legible?

V. Are all reports/tests/procedures initialed (all entries) by the physician after being reviewed?

SECTION

2

MEDICAL DOCUMENTATION

Introduction

Medical office documentation has changed a great deal in the last few years, largely due to the implementation of managed care. In previous traditional office settings, the only workers with access to a patient's chart were the physician and office staff. Now, because of managed care, a patient's medical record is reviewed on a regular basis by various managed care groups. Insurance reviewers check to ensure that charts are complete, accurate, and organized. Section 1 of this book provides a sample of what types of information an insurance company looks for when doing a chart review. Each of the sample charts in this section was specifically developed to adhere to the latest guidelines set forth by many new managed care plans.

To efficiently perform the vital function of charting, several basic principles should be reviewed.

The first principle concerns the legal aspects of medical documentation. The medical chart is a legal document that can be used in a court of law. The need for accuracy and neatness cannot be stressed enough. Medical professional liability cases have been lost due to inaccurate, incomplete, or indecipherable documentation practices.

The second principle regards confidentiality. Information that is given to the physician and/or staff is considered "privileged communication." This means no member of the physician's office staff can release any information about a patient without the written authorization (signature) of a patient, unless the records are subpoenaed by a court of law.

Make sure that when obtaining information from a patient you do so in a private setting, which will help alleviate the possibility of someone overhearing information that should be kept confidential. You also must guard against the possibility of a breach of confidentiality while using the computer or word processor. The monitor should be kept out of the scope of vision of patients and others who should not have access to confidential information.

Tactfulness is yet another principle that should be followed when obtaining medical information. It is important to not only think of *what* questions to ask a patient, but just as important *how* they are going to be asked. Overt facial expressions should be discouraged. Passing judgment on a patient because of his or her views or lifestyle also should be avoided.

The following charts provide the reader with simple questions to ask for various situations that will arise in the medical office—everything from progress notes to documenting outside procedures will be included in this section.

How to Use the Charts

IN AN OFFICE SITUATION:

1. All charts should be reviewed with the physician, prior to implementation.

2. If any adjustments need to be made, they should be written in the modification section that appears at the bottom of the chart.

3. The physician will then need to sign the chart to show that he or she agrees with the format the chart follows.

IN A CLASSROOM ENVIRONMENT:

1. Charts should be reviewed by the instructor prior to implementation in the classroom.

2. Any adjustments that need to be made should be written in the modification section that appears at the bottom of the chart. (Make adjustments in pencil so they may be erased if future changes occur.)

3. There is no need for the instructor to sign her or his name on the chart, since it will be used in practice situations only.

Note:

Some of the charts refer to another section of this book. An example of this is the Chief Complaint Chart. To begin documentation of the complaint, answer questions 1–3. Question 4 instructs you to turn to the appropriate assessment chart that corresponds with the symptoms of the patient. Once the assessment portion of the complaint is completed, refer back to the Chief Complaint Chart to finish documentation.

CHIEF COMPLAINT

A chief complaint is a brief description of what is wrong with the patient. The opening phrase should be concise, using the patient's own words. Standard abbreviations should be used whenever possible. The chart listed below provides the necessary information for documenting a chief complaint.

EXPANDED CHIEF COMPLAINT

Parts of the Complaint	Description
1. Today's date	
2. Nature of complaint	A brief description of what is wrong with the patient. (Use the patient's own words in this part of the complaint.)
3. Date of onset or duration	When did the patient first notice symptoms, or how long have they persisted?
4. Developmental questions	These can be found in the assessment portion of the book, underneath the complaint with which the symptoms correspond.
5. Any self-remedies (Did they help?)	Has the patient taken any medications or administered any treatment to help alleviate symptoms?
6. In addition to #5, what other things make symptoms better or worse?	i.e., lying down, standing up, etc.
7. List medications currently being taken by the patient	All prescribed medications and non-prescribed. (This will have a bearing on what the physician can prescribe for the patient.)
8. Update the patient's status on drug allergies	Never assume that just because the patient's chart is not flagged, that he or she does not have any drug allergies. Use the initials *NKDA* in cases where the patient has no known drug allergies.
9. Exit signature	First initial and last name
10. Physician's initials	

Any Modifications:_____

_____

_____

_____

_____

_____

Physician's Approval:_____

EXPANDED COMPLAINT

Pros:	Helps the assistant anticipate what types of necessary tray setups, procedures, etc. the physician might want to perform prior to examining the patient. Gives the physician better insight into what issues he or she might be dealing with. Saves the physician's time, overall.
Cons:	Ties up the assistant for a greater amount of time. Increases the amount of paper in the chart. Patients may not reveal everything to the physician, because the patient has already discussed it with the assistant.

EXAMPLE

04-07-xx: Pt c/o an intermittent HA x 4 days. "The pain starts in the back of my head and radiates to the front of my head, above my L eyebrow." + dizziness, − neck pain, + N/V, some visual disturbances during the pain episodes. Pt taking Tylenol. (Little relief.) "Pain never goes away completely." No current prescribed meds. NKDA. H. Neff (BT)

BRIEF EXPANDED COMPLAINT

Pros:	Gives enough information so the assistant can anticipate what to set up. Saves the assistant's time. Frees up some paper space.
Cons:	Makes the physician ask more questions.

EXAMPLE

04-07-xx: Pt c/o of HA x 4 days. + dizziness, + N/V, some visual difficulties during episodes. H. Neff (BT)

BRIEF COMPLAINT

Pros:	Keeps the patient from revealing his or her full complaint to both the physician and assistant. Provides a greater amount of patient confidentiality. Saves a great deal of the assistant's time. Frees up paper space in the chart. (Keep in mind that the majority of the physician's notes are transcribed.)
Cons:	Assistant's anticipation skills will be weakened. Requires more work for the physician. Could extend the amount of time the patient is detained.

EXAMPLE

04-07-xx: CC: HA x 4 days. H. Neff (BT)

FOLLOW-UP APPOINTMENTS/PROGRESS NOTES

Patients will often be asked to return for a follow-up appointment after an initial visit. This can be a one-time follow-up or a series of follow-ups. Listening skills are critical in these types of visits. Patients might intentionally, or inadvertently, say things that can be significant for both their medical progress or for future legal purposes. The chart below lists important information that should be included in a progress note:

PROGRESS NOTES

Parts of the Progress Notes	Descriptions or Facts
1. Date	
2. Final diagnosis from last appointment or why patient is here today. (If diagnostic testing was performed during the last visit, attach the results to the front of the patient's chart.)	Some physicians will want this listed but many will just look at the last entry to get this information. (Assistant should still be aware as to why the pt is coming in.)
3. Current symptoms	List current symptoms the patient has to date. List any changes as well.
4. Were home care instructions followed? (If not, why?)	Examples: Did patient take all of his or her medication, did they change bandages, follow up with a specialist, etc. (very important for legal purposes).
5. Exit signature	First initial, last name
6. Physician's initials	

EXAMPLE

6-4-xx: Pt here for a F/U from 5-25-xx. Sutures are scheduled to be removed today. Dressing was dry and clean. No erythema, drainage or edema. Pt took all of antibiotic and followed all home care instructions. "Thumb is still a little sore but pain is tolerable." M. Thompson (BT)

Any Modifications: _____

_____

_____

_____

_____

_____

Physician's Approval:_____

DOCUMENTING MEDICATIONS

The administration of medication is an important task that is routinely done in the medical office. Equally important is the documentation of such medication. To understand how to properly document these procedures, you must first understand a very important rule. NEVER DOCUMENT A MEDICATION THAT YOU DID NOT PREPARE OR ADMINISTER! The person who prepares the medication should administer it as well as document it. The person who documents the medication is the one who will be held accountable should a lawsuit arise. The chart below lists the information that should be included when documenting medications.

DOCUMENTATION OF MEDICATIONS

Information to Be Documented	Descriptions or Facts
1. Today's date	
2. Name of medication	Write out the entire name so there is no misunderstanding.
3. Strength of medication (dose given)	Many medications come in various strengths; be specific.
4. Route of administration	IM, Sub Q, ID, buccally, orally, or sublingually
5. Site used	Where did you administer the medication, i.e., the deltoid, gluteal muscle, back of arm, etc.?
6. Name of doctor who ordered the medication	Who authorized the medication? If ordered by someone outside the facility, be sure to attach the written order to the chart. This will comply with federal, state, and CLIA/COLA guidelines. (This applies to all procedures.)
If immunization, include the following information: **(May have a special form that is part of the consent form that will answer these questions.)**	
7. Manufacturer's name	Many manufacturers make the same drug— BE SPECIFIC!
8. Lot #	If there is a problem with the medication, it is important to know the lot # so you can inform the manufacturer. The opposite also holds true.
9. Expiration date	Never give a medication that has reached or passed its expiration date.
10. Name and address of physician	Some states require this for legal purposes. An address stamp saves time.
For all medications:	
11. Any problems encountered	i.e., any swelling at the injection site, etc.
12. Any educational material handed out	i.e., immunizations, certain hormone shots, etc.

(continued on next page)

DOCUMENTATION OF MEDICATIONS *(continued from previous page)*

13. Physician's initials
_____

Any Modifications: _____
_____
_____
_____
_____
_____

Physician's Approval:_____

EXAMPLE # 1

02-13-xx: Gave 0.5 mℓ of Adult Tetanus Toxoid, IM, R Deltoid per Dr. Kent Smith, 2252 Oak Street, Columbus, OH, 43221. SKB Lot #246 Exp 2-Yr. M. Paisly (KS)

EXAMPLE # 2

02-15-xx: Gave 0.5 mℓ of allergy serum, Sub Q, R Arm per Dr. Smith. Small wheal formed about the size of a dime at the injection site following the injection.
+ Redness, + Edema. Site is sore and tender. − Respiratory Sx. Applied ice to the area. Informed doctor of reaction. Dr would like the dose to be reduced to 0.4 mℓ next visit. M. Heller. (KS)

DOCUMENTING PRESCRIPTIONS

Writing and documenting prescriptions are very important tasks in the physician's office. The documentation of prescriptions will be addressed in this section. To review how to write a prescription, turn to Section 6 under Parts of the Prescription.

Every prescription must be double checked before calling it into the pharmacy, and double checked again with the pharmacist. Use abbreviations whenever possible in this section and pay close attention to detail. The chart below is useful for documenting prescriptions:

CHARTING PRESCRIPTIONS

Information to Be Documented	Descriptions or Facts
1. Today's date	
2. Pharmacy's name, location, and phone # and pharmacist's name	This will help alleviate any misunderstandings as to which pharmacy was called.
3. Name of medication	Write out the entire name so there are no misunderstandings.
4. Strength of medication	Many medications come in different strengths.
5. Amount to be dispensed	When it applies
6. Special instructions	This lists how much is to be taken, how often, and how to take it, i.e., before or after meals, at bedtime, when symptoms occur, and how long to take it.
7. Any refills	
8. Who ordered the prescription	Which doctor in the practice ordered the medication.
9. Exit signature	First initial, last name
10. Physician's initials	Doctor should initial all prescriptions that are called into a pharmacy.

Any Modifications:

_____

_____

_____

_____

_____

Physician's Approval:_____

EXAMPLE

6-09-xx: Called in Rx to Howell's Pharmacy, S. High Street, 555-0099. Spoke to pharmacist Bob Tucker: Amoxicillin, 250 mg, #30, Sig 1 cap. tid x 10 days per Dr. Jones. M. Brown (EJ)

CHARTING IN-HOUSE PROCEDURES

Documentation of the procedures that are performed is an important function in the medical office. The chart below lists the information that should be included when documenting in-house procedures.

PROCEDURE DOCUMENTATION

Information to Be Documented	Descriptions or Facts
1. Today's date	
2. Name or names of procedures	i.e., EKG, UA, C&S, CBC, etc.
3. Name of physician ordering procedure	
4. If procedure is blood test list:	From where did you collect the specimen? How much did you collect, and what procedure did you use to collect the specimen (i.e., vacutainer, syringe, butterfly, etc.)? List any failed attempts.
5. Where lab tests were sent	i.e., Roche, Met-Path, etc.
6. List acquisition number when it applies.	i.e., this is the number the lab uses to identify the specimen.
7. List anatomical locations when referring to other types of procedures.	i.e., chest Xray PA and lateral; sutures removed from R Foot
8. Did patient experience any problems during the procedure?	i.e., passed out, fainting, N/V, etc.
9. Any special instructions given to patient	
10. Exit signature	First initial, last name
11. Physician's initials	Many insurance companies want the physician to initial all entries made in the chart. Physician needs to confirm that his or her orders were carried out.

Any Modifications: _____

_____

_____

_____

_____

Physician's Approval:_____

EXAMPLE

01-22-xx: Order (physician writes)	Procedure
CBC	*Venipuncture of L antecubital space.*
Chem 12	*1 Lavender & 2*
Thyroid Panel	*Red Tops sent to Roche Labs. #78902,*
	per Dr. Jones, no complications
	during or following procedure. M. Harris (EJ)

Whenever it applies, document procedures performed into the appropriate logs, i.e., Urine Dipstick Log, Xray Log, Lab Log.

CHARTING OUTSIDE PROCEDURES

There may be occasions where it will be necessary to refer patients to outside facilities. Good documentation for these entries will be important for informative and legal purposes. Always check with the insurance company regarding pre-certification requirements before scheduling any outside procedure. Refer to Section 12 in this book for a sample Pre-Certification Form and a Plan Information Form. If the insurance company does give pre-approval for an outside procedure, be sure to document it. Listed below is a useful chart to assist you in documenting these types of procedures.

DOCUMENTATION OF OUTSIDE PROCEDURES

Information to Be Documented	Descriptions or Facts
1. Today's date	
2. Name of procedure or test to be done	Reference purposes
3. Name of facility and location	Reference purposes
4. Date and time of procedure	Reference purposes
5. Who ordered the procedure	Legal purposes
6. Who you spoke to	In case there are any problems, speak directly to the person who set up the exam.
7. Special instructions	Is any special preparation involved prior to having the procedure, i.e., special clothing and/or paperwork to be completed?
8. Confirmation to patient	Show that this information was confirmed with the patient.
9. Exit signature	First initial, last name
10. Physician's initials	To confirm to the physician that the procedure did get ordered. (Many insurance companies want all entries to be initialed by the physician.)

Any Modifications: _____

_____

_____

_____

_____

_____

Physician's Approval:_____

02-22-xx: Obtained pre-approval from Sandy at Cigna to schedule the patient for a uterine ultrasound. Certification # 55678F J. Thomas (JS)

02-23-xx: Scheduled uterine ultrasound at Riverside General, Room 2A in lower level of hospital for 2-24-xx at 9:00 a.m. per Dr. Sound. Spoke with Cindy: "Pt is to come with a full bladder. Instruct to drink 6-8 glasses of water before arriving for test." Called and confirmed this information with the patient. J. Thomas (JS)

TELEPHONE TRIAGE

Triaging of phone calls is difficult because of the fine line issue. The person doing the assessment not only has to determine what might be wrong with the patient, but also might have to give the patient instructions based upon the nature of the complaint. This is difficult because it throws the assistant into a role that is very close to diagnosing and/or prescribing.

The ultimate situation in office telephone triaging would be if the physician could triage all of his or her own calls. This would be a wonderful scenario, however, it is not practical. Physicians have a hard enough time adhering to a schedule without this added task. Before setting up office telephone guidelines, the physician and his or her staff must consider the possible medicolegal issues, as well as specific guidelines set forth by the insurance companies with which the physician associates.

The following is a list of suggestions that, if implemented, could help reduce the possibility of potential lawsuits.

1. Decide how many telephone lines will be needed based on the amount of calls coming into the office.

2. Decide how many people will be needed to handle the lines.

3. Decide which personnel is capable of handling the task, i.e., nurse, physician's assistant, or medical assistant. Keep in mind state policies and insurance company regulations. Past experience also should be a factor.

4. Incorporate a telephone triage manual that best reflects the philosophies of the physician(s). (Section 3 of this book provides a section on telephone triage.)

5. Have the staff you chose to do the telephone triaging complete a training program to learn office policies and the triage manual.

6. Implement a method to evaluate communication skills and reading comprehension of the triage personnel.

7. Review telephone triage standards whenever a new physician is hired or the physician becomes associated with a new managed care plan.

8. Reassess new options such as the number of telephone lines coming into the office, the type of telephone system used, and the number of people handling the calls, as the practice grows.

9. Document employee training and record in the employee's record.

The telephone triage chart that follows provides questions that should be asked in any telephone triage situation. Question five on the triage chart requires the user to turn to the assessment chart that corresponds with the symptoms of the patient.

Many phone calls that come into the medical office will require the assistant to set up an appointment, however, in some cases home treatment may be sufficient. It is important not to vary from this chart, as this will venture into the territory of prescribing. Before suggesting any OTC (over-the-counter) medications, read the OTC instructions.

Some medical offices want assistants to offer all patients who call an opportunity for an appointment. This is not always an option, but it is a good rule of thumb to follow in offices where the opportunity affords itself.

In any situation where the patient requests to speak with the physician, or there is fear or apprehension, the call should be directed to the physician.

Note:

All telephone triage documentation must be reviewed by the physician and initialed. When a complaint arises that is not listed on any of the assessment charts, the physician should be consulted before making any decisions.

TELEPHONE TRIAGE	
Information to Be Documented	**Descriptions or Facts**
1. Today's date and time of call	
2. General complaint	Why the patient called
3. Date of onset	When did symptoms begin?
4. Time of onset	If injuries occurred as a result of an accident in which legal issues may be raised (industrial or vehicular).
5. Developmental questions	These can be found in Section 3 of this book, underneath the complaint with which the symptoms correspond.
6. Any self-remedies	Has the patient taken any medications or administered any treatment to help alleviate symptoms?
7. List instructions given to patient	Was the patient set up for an appointment, encouraged to call the EMS, or given home care instructions?
8. Document refusal to follow instructions	i.e., the patient's refusal to follow instructions could be significant in a professional liability suit.
9. Exit signature	First initial, last name
10. Physician's initials	This is to show that the physician was made aware of the call. Many insurance companies require the physician to initial all entries made in the chart.

Any Modifications:

_____

_____

_____

_____

_____

Physician's Approval:_____

EXAMPLE

06-12-xx: TC: 2:15 p.m. Pt called to say that she was having chest pain. "Pain starts in the center of my chest and radiates to my left side." Pain started 30 minutes ago and has not subsided. + SOB, − N/V, + dizziness + tingling in left arm and hand. Pt has no personal Hx of heart disease but father died five years ago of a heart attack. No other Sx. Instructed pt to call 911 and have the EMS come out to do an evaluation. Pt refused to follow instructions. Pt wants husband to drive her to Riverside General ER. Informed pt of possible consequences. Pt still insisted on going to ER. Will call Riverside General and let them know that pt is on her way. P. Hinson (℘)

SECTION

3

MEDICAL ASSESSMENT

Introduction

Assessment in the physician's office is uniquely different from the type of assessment which takes place in a hospital setting or in an extended care facility.

In the hospital setting, the patient goes for long intervals without seeing the physician. The nurse's assessment skills must be thorough and in-depth to bring the physician up to date on the patient's progress.

However, assessment in the physician's office is quite distinct. Patients who are scheduled for an appointment with the physician will ultimately be evaluated by the physician.

Health care personnel employed by a physician's office are still involved in the assessment procedure, however, how detailed that assessment will be is determined by the physician. Workers perform initial assessments, which occur before the patient sees the physician, and they also perform telephone assessments.

In general, the initial assessment has to provide enough information to prepare the assistant and the physician for the patient's exam. The assistant has to be able to instruct the patient about how to disrobe, as well as what preliminary preparations are necessary. Providing the physician with initial assessment information makes the assistant's job easier because it gives the physician an opportunity to review past findings to see if any patterns might be developing.

Telephone assessment involves more than just asking questions. The assistant must have the ability to know how to direct the patient according to his or her symptoms. As previously discussed under Telephone Triage in Section 2, it is critical that the telephone triage manual represents the physician's philosophies.

The following section offers general assessment questions that can be used in both office and telephone situations. It also lists possible procedures the physician might want set up prior to examining the patient, based upon the patient's complaint. The final portion of the chart lists telephone instructions for the patient.

These charts are helpful for students who are just learning assessment skills. They also provide students with anticipation skills and are excellent aids for assistants who are already working in the field.

When using the charts in the field, they must first be reviewed with the physician. Make any changes that need to be made in the modification section. Be sure to have the physician sign the chart after reviewing it. This will show that he or she agrees with the protocol on the chart and that he or she will be assured that physician's orders are followed. It also will help to promote consistency in the office among staff members.

If some charts in this section do not reflect the criteria of your office, a blank General Complaint Form can be found in Section 12. This chart can be duplicated and personalized to meet the needs of your office. Be sure to have the physician approve the chart by signing his or her name on the Physician's Approval line.

Important Information
About the Charts

The general complaint charts that follow are divided into three columns.

The first column lists assessment questions that should be asked in both office and telephone situations.

The second column lists special equipment, supplies, or procedures that the physician might want set up based on the patient's symptoms. This column is designed to help the student with anticipation skills, but probably will not be necessary for the veteran assistant. Even though procedures will vary from one physician to another, it is wise to teach the student to think ahead. *Never run any test or perform any procedure without a direct order from the physician.* Setting up the procedure ahead of time will save time later if the physician does in fact order that procedure.

The third column contains instructions that can be given to the patient based on his or her complaint. The third column is shaded for easy visual identification. A common rule of thumb should be followed in triage situations—offer all patients the opportunity for an appointment. If the patient declines, the instructions that have been pre-approved by the physician may then be given. Be sure to document if an appointment was offered and whether or not the patient decided to accept or decline it.

The abbreviation and code key that follows the assessment instructions provides the reader with a description of all of the abbreviations and codes used in the assessment charts.

The bottom of each chart lists possible disrobing instructions and the vital signs that may need to be taken, based on the patient's complaint. Additional telephone instructions for the patient may be included as well.

After reviewing the charts with the physician, the assistant may want to make adjustments in the modification section. Remember to have the physician sign his or her name at the bottom of the charts.

Over-the-counter medications that were pre-approved by the physician for the patient's use at home can be written on the blank Over-the-Counter Adult Chart, found in Section 12 of this book. Also found in this section is the blank Over-the-Counter Pediatric Chart. Notice that both charts list only the drug categories. This allows the physician the opportunity to provide the top three medications he or she feels is appropriate for each category. Section 6 of this book also charts the leading over-the-counter medications. This information may aid the assistant and physician in filling in the blank OTC charts.

How to Use the Charts

1. The assessment chart is always used in conjunction with another chart, i.e., the Chief Complaint Form, Telephone Triage Form, etc.

2. After using the preliminary chart, the assistant should ask the questions in Column 1.

3. Some charts will have a notation under the question (the assistant should read all questions before making any decisions). It is important that the assistant ask all questions before making any decisions or he or she might miss an important symptom and provide the patient with the wrong instructions.

4. If the patient is calling on the telephone, the assistant should give the instructions listed in Column 3 that correlate with the patient's symptoms. If the patient has more than one symptom and needs to be seen by the physician, the assistant should choose the most serious response that the patient answered "yes" to, i.e., if the patient answered "yes" to three different symptoms and the responses in column 3 say SDA, (24), or STAT, the assistant should give the instructions for a STAT visit, as it is the most serious of the three.

5. If the assistant is questioning the patient in the office, use the instructions in Column 2 entitled Possible Procedures. This means the procedure may have to be set up. As mentioned previously, *never run any test without a direct order from the physician.*

6. Before suggesting any OTC medications in Column 3, the assistant should read and understand the OTC medication instructions, found in Section 6 of this book.

7. The assistant should be sure to return to the original chart he or she was using before completing documentation, i.e., the Chief Complaint Chart or Telephone Triage Chart.

ABBREVIATION AND CODE KEY

The following list has been specially designed for use in the assessment section. It illustrates standard abbreviations and symbols that can be found in the next section, as well as directional codes that also are displayed in the assessment section. These codes are designed to provide the assistant with specific directions for the patient.

CODE KEY

DIRECTIONAL CODES

Code	Description
1. (EMS)	Patient should contact the emergency medical services.
2. (STAT)	Patient should be seen in the office as soon as possible.
3. (SDA)	Same day appointment
4. (24)	Patient should be seen within a 24-hour period.
5. (48)	Patient should be seen within a 48-hour period.
6. (ER)	Patient should go directly to an emergency facility.
7. (WK)	Patient should be seen within the week.

SYMBOLS

Code	Description	Code	Description
>	Greater Than	+	Positive
<	Less Than	−	Negative
#	Number	=	Equals
×	Times	*	A place for the assistant to personalize notes
$\bar{c}$	With	$\bar{s}$	Without
♀	Female	♂	Male
↓	Decreased	↑	Increased

ABBREVIATIONS

Abbreviation	Definition
ASAP	As Soon As Possible
bid	Twice a Day
BM	Bowel Movement
BP	Blood Pressure
CBC	Complete Blood Count
CC	Chief Complaint
Chem	Chemistry
c/o	Complains Of
C&S	Culture and Sensitivity
Dr	Doctor
ECG and EKG	Electrocardiogram
EDC	Expected, Estimated Date of Confinement
e.g.	For example
EMS	Emergency Medical Services (British)
ENT	Ear, Nose, Throat
ER	Emergency Room
F	Fahrenheit
F/U	Follow-Up
GC	Gonorrhea Culture
GI	Gastrointestinal
gravida, grav	A pregnant woman; pregnancy
GTT	Glucose Tolerance Test
HA	Headache
HC	Head Circumference
Hct and HCT	Hematocrit
H&H	Hematocrit and Hemoglobin
hrs	Hours
HT	Height
Hx	History
ID	Intradermal
i.e.	That is
IM	Intramuscular, Intermuscular
KOH	Potassium-Hydroxide
L	Left
LMP	Last Menstrual Period
ml	Milliliter
mg	Milligram
NC	No Change
N/O	No Complaints
NKDA	No Known Drug Allergies
N/V	Nausea and Vomiting

(continued on following page)

ABBREVIATIONS *(continued from previous page)*

Abbreviation	Definition
OTC	Over-the-Counter
oz	Ounce
P	Pulse
PA	Posteroanterior
para	Number of viable births
pre-	Before
pt	Patient
q	Every
R	Right or Respiration
re	Regarding
Rx	Medication, drugs
Sig	Label; write
SOB	Shortness of breath
SPF	Sun Protection Factor
STAT	Immediately
STD	Sexually Transmitted Disease
Sub Q	Subcutaneous
Sx and sx	Symptom(s)
T	Temperature
tab	Tablet
TC	Telephone Call
tid	Three times a day
TPR	Temperature, Pulse, Respiration
tsp	Teaspoon; teaspoonful
UA	Urinalysis
URI	Upper Respiratory Infection
UTI	Urinary Tract Infection
WT	Weight

GENERAL COMPLAINT: ABDOMINAL PAIN

COLUMN 1	COLUMN 2	COLUMN 3
QUESTIONS (Ask all questions before making any decisions)	**POSSIBLE PROCEDURES** (If patient is in the office)	**TELEPHONE TRIAGE**
1. Location, intensity and pain pattern (List on a scale from 1-10)		
If pain is severe, constant, or combined with other symptoms:	Provide comfort measures for the patient	(STAT)
2. Fever		
If T is >101° F or has lasted > 24 hrs:	Provide comfort measures for the patient	(STAT)
If T is < 101° F or has lasted < 24 hrs:	Provide comfort measures for the patient	(SDA) (When combined with other symptoms)
3. Nausea or Vomiting	Provide emesis basin	
If patient appears dehydrated or symptoms are combined with severe pain:	If patient is thirsty do not give anything to drink until the physician okays it. (Possible surgery)	(STAT)
(Dehydration signs are on the next page)		
If symptoms are mild and abdominal pain is light:	Comfort measures should be provided	Give patient instructions on how to stay hydrated Pt should notify office if Sx worsen (Hydration instructions are on the next page)
4. Diarrhea		
If > 5-6 watery stools in 12 hrs:	Possible stool cultures and rectal exam	(SDA)
If < 5-6 watery stools in 12 hrs and other Sx are mild:		Clear liquids for 24 hrs as Sx subside, start on Brat diet (see next page) and OTC antidiarrheal (check with physician)
5. Last bowel movement		

(continued on following page)

GENERAL COMPLAINT: ABDOMINAL PAIN *(continued from previous page)*

COLUMN 1	COLUMN 2	COLUMN 3
QUESTIONS	POSSIBLE PROCEDURES	TELEPHONE TRIAGE
(Ask all questions before making any decisions)	(If patient is in the office)	
6. Any blood, pus, or mucus in stools?	Possible stool cultures and rectal exam	(SDA)
7. Any vaginal symptoms (female)?	Possible pelvic exam and STD cultures	(SDA)-(24)
8. Any penile symptoms (male)?	Possible STD cultures	(SDA)-(24)
9. Any urinary symptoms?	Possible UA and & C&S	(SDA)
10. Any trauma to abdomen?	Possible abdominal Xrays	(STAT)
11. If pain is mild and intermittent with no other symptoms:		Take OTC pain reliever. (Check with physician.) If pain continues >24 hrs or worsens, contact office immediately.

Vitals: BP & T

Disrobing Instructions: If Sx are above waist (waist up), if Sx are below waist (completely)

Diarrhea Protocol (Clear Liquid Diet) For the first 24 hours, the patient should only take in clear liquids, i.e., flat sodas, weak tea, and Jell-O. Can give Pedialyte to infants. Liquids should be offered a minimum of every 2 hours. Brat diet can be instituted after the first 24 hours and after the diarrhea subsides. (Bananas, rice, applesauce, and dry toast for approximately 48 hours.) Once diarrhea completely stops, patient may resume normal diet. If symptoms reoccur, patient should schedule an appointment.

Dehydration Signs: Dry mouth, no urine output in last 8-10 hours (if urine is dark in color and has a strong odor), listlessness, dry mouth, sunken eyeballs, or absence of tears. *Infants should be seen right away, because they can dehydrate quickly.*

Rehydration Instructions: Offer fluids as often as possible; encourage patient to drink fluids such as Gatorade in adults and Pedialyte in infants. If symptoms persist greater than _____ hours patient should notify office ASAP.

Any Modifications: _____

_____

Physician's Approval: _____

GENERAL COMPLAINT: BACK PAIN

COLUMN 1	COLUMN 2	COLUMN 3
QUESTIONS	**POSSIBLE PROCEDURES**	**TELEPHONE TRIAGE**
(Ask all questions before making any decisions)	(If patient is in the office)	
1. Location and intensity (List pain on a scale from 1-10)		
2. Any urinary Sx?	Possible UA and C&S	(SDA)
3. Any abdominal pain?		If severe (SDA)
4. If pain is in mid-back, ask pt if any cough or cold symptoms are present. If so:	Possible chest Xray	(SDA)
5. Any recent injuries to back?	Possible Xray	(SDA)
6. Any neck pain?	Possible Xray	(STAT)
7. Tingling in other parts of the body?	Possible Xray	(STAT)
If neck pain or tingling follows an injury, do not move pt		(EMS)
8. Any vaginal symptoms (female)?	Possible pelvic tray and STD cultures	(SDA)-(24)
9. Any penile symptoms (male)?	Set up for STD cultures	(SDA)-(24)
10. Last BM and texture (if abnormal)	Possible stool culture	(SDA)-(24)
11. Fever >101° F		(SDA)-(24)
12. If pain is mild and does not appear to involve other organs:		Apply heat to area and take an OTC pain reliever. Notify office if pain worsens.

(continued on following page)

GENERAL COMPLAINT: BACK PAIN *(continued from previous page)*

COLUMN 1	COLUMN 2	COLUMN 3
QUESTIONS	POSSIBLE PROCEDURES	TELEPHONE TRIAGE
(Ask all questions before making any decisions)	**(If patient is in the office)**	
If pain is severe or appears to involve other organs,		
i.e., kidneys or lungs, spinal cord, etc.	Possible Xray for areas involved	(SDA)

Vitals: BP & T

Disrobing Instructions: If Sx above waist, (waist up), Sx below waist (completely)

Any Modifications:

_____

_____

_____

_____

_____

Physician's Approval: _____

GENERAL COMPLAINT: BURNS

COLUMN 1 QUESTIONS (Ask all questions before making any decisions)	COLUMN 2 POSSIBLE PROCEDURES (If patient is in the office)	COLUMN 3 TELEPHONE TRIAGE
1. Nature of burn		
2. Type of burn (chemical, thermal, or electrical)	Provide comfort measures until physician sees patient	Follow criteria listed below, based on what type of burn the patient has.
3. Location and diameter of burn		If burn appears on the feet, hands, face, buttocks, or genital region (STAT)
4. If burn falls under the following criteria:	Provide comfort measures until physician sees patient	(STAT)
A. Burn looks infected		
B. Skin is charred		
C. Suspect child abuse (pediatric patient)		
D. Skin is open or coming off		
E. Blisters are greater than ____ inches		
F. Intense pain		
G. Patient is elderly or very young		
5. Amount of pain	Provide comfort measures	If pain is severe, patient should be seen right away.
6. Any breathing problems?	Provide comfort measures (Get physician ASAP)	If severe, call EMS. If not (STAT).

Immediate Response Instructions:

Thermal burn: Flush or immerse area intermittently in ice water or cool tap water for a minimum of 10 minutes. If area cannot be immersed or flushed, apply ice to area.

Chemical burn: Remove clothing and flush skin thoroughly with water until chemical is completely removed from the skin. If eyes are affected, flush skin with steady stream of water for a minimum of 10-15 minutes.

Electrical burn: Apply cold compresses to area immediately. If there are any respiratory symptoms or if the patient stops breathing, call the local EMS immediately.

All electrical burns should be referred to the ER, as there could be internal damage not visible to the naked eye.

(continued on following page)

GENERAL COMPLAINT: BURNS *(continued from previous page)*

Home Care Management Instructions: If burn area is small (< quarter), 1st degree, does not follow any symptoms or conditions listed in #4, and is not located in any of the areas listed in #3, home care instructions may be given: Patient may continue to immerse burn in water or apply cold compresses, take OTC analgesic and follow up by calling the office within 1-2 hours following burn. Do not instruct patient to apply topical ointments or sprays unless directed by the physician. Notify the office immediately if there are any signs of infection.

Sunburn: The best defense against sunburn is prevention. All patients should be encouraged to use a sunscreen with a sun protection factor (SPF) of 15 or greater. Limit sun exposure time and wear proper clothing. If patient does get sunburned, apply cold wet compresses to the area and a lubricant that the physician approves, i.e., Vaseline, etc. Do not attempt to pop blisters. If blisters appear, the patient should be seen. Patient may want to take an OTC-analgesic if the pain is strong. Notify the office immediately if there are any signs of infection.

Vitals: BP, T, P & R

Any Modifications: _____

_____

_____

_____

_____

_____

Physician's Approval: _____

GENERAL COMPLAINT: CHEST PAIN

COLUMN 1	COLUMN 2	COLUMN 3
QUESTIONS	POSSIBLE PROCEDURES	TELEPHONE TRIAGE
(If pain is associated with any of the Sx in #2-7, call the EMS.)	(If patient is in the office)	
1. Exact location and intensity of pain		
If pain is mild and intermittent with no other Sx:	Set up for possible EKG	(SDA)
If pain is severe and persists for > than 2 minutes or other Sx are present:	Set up for EKG, notify physician ASAP	(EMS)
2. Shortness of breath?	Set up for EKG, notify physician ASAP	(EMS)
3. Does pain radiate to any other part of the body? (L arm, jaw, neck, or back) If so:	Set up for EKG, notify physician ASAP	(EMS)
4. Any Hx of heart problems?	Set up for EKG, notify physician ASAP	(EMS)
5. Nausea or vomiting? If so, give patient emesis basin.	Set up for EKG, notify physician ASAP	(EMS)
6. Lightheadedness or dizziness?	Stay with patient. Set up for EKG, notify physician ASAP	(EMS)
7. Discoloration to skin?		(EMS)
8. Indigestion (if pain appears more epigastric with no other chest-related symptoms)?		OTC antacid. If Sx persist or worsen F/U immediately with office.

Vitals: BP, P & R. Put patient in room with access to crash tray or cart. Be prepared to call EMS if necessary.

Disrobing Instructions: Waist up

(continued on following page)

GENERAL COMPLAINT: CHEST PAIN *(continued from previous page)*

Any Modifications: _____

_____

_____

_____

_____

_____

Physician's Approval: _____

GENERAL COMPLAINT: COLD SYMPTOMS (Sore Throat, Congestion, Cough)

COLUMN 1 QUESTIONS (Ask all questions before making any decisions)	COLUMN 2 POSSIBLE PROCEDURES (If patient is in the office)	COLUMN 3 TELEPHONE TRIAGE
1. Runny or stuffy nose?	Nasal speculum	OTC cold formula
(record color)		
If discharge is thick and colored:		(SDA)–(24)
2. Sore or scratchy throat?	Tongue depressor and pen light	Warm salt water gargles (1/4 tsp to 4 oz warm water)
		Leading OTC pain reliever
If swollen or patches of pus:	Possible rapid strep test or throat culture	(SDA)
3. Ear pain or pressure?	Otoscope, ear curette	(SDA)
(document any drainage)		
4. Headache?	Possible cervical spine films	OTC pain reliever
(if severe)	Turn down lights in exam room	(SDA)
Sinus pressure or neck pain?	Possible sinus films	(SDA)
5. Swollen glands?		(SDA)
6. Cough?		OTC cough formula
(if cough is hard or productive)	Possible chest Xray or sputum analysis	(SDA)
7. Facial pain or pressure?		OTC decongestant
(if severe)	Possible sinus films	(SDA)–(24)
8. Eyes sensitive to light?	Turn down lights in exam room	(SDA)–(24)
9. Fever (list route and how high)?		
(if > 100° F or has lasted > 2 days)		(SDA)
10. Neck pain or stiffness?	Possible lumbar puncture	(STAT), ASAP

(continued on following page)

3

GENERAL COMPLAINT: COLD SYMPTOMS (SORE THROAT, CONGESTION, COUGH) *(continued from previous page)*

Vitals: All

Disrobing Instructions: If Sx above neck (none); if cough is present or patient complains of chest pressure (waist up); if patient has swollen glands (totally).

Trays: None

Any Modifications: _____

_____

_____

_____

_____

Physician's Approval: _____

GENERAL COMPLAINT: EYE DISORDERS

COLUMN 1 QUESTIONS (Ask all questions before making any decisions)	COLUMN 2 POSSIBLE PROCEDURES (If patient is in the office)	COLUMN 3 TELEPHONE TRIAGE
1. Nature of complaint		
2. Does patient remember injuring eye? (if so, how)	Do visual acuity (if possible) Cover affected eye (eye tray)	(SDA); cover affected eye
3. Any swelling or redness?	Repeat instructions for # 2	If severe (SDA) If Sx are minor, follow home care instructions listed below
4. Any foreign object in eye?	Do not attempt to remove. Cover eye and wait for instructions. Set up eye tray.	(SDA)
5. Is skin red around eye?	Repeat instructions for #2	(SDA)
6. Any drainage coming from eye?	Set up eye tray and do visual acuity; possible culture	If drainage is thick, colored, or eye is matted shut, (SDA). May apply warm washcloth over eye to help open. If drainage is clear, follow home care instructions listed below.
7. Any itching (if yes)		(SDA)
8. Any Hx of eye problems in the past?		Possible home care instructions
9. Any cold symptoms?	Make patient comfortable	If mild, give OTC cold formula instructions. If Sx severe (SDA)
10. Any fever?	Make patient comfortable	(SDA)
11. Any associated allergy symptoms?	Make patient comfortable	If severe (SDA) If mild, OTC allergy medicine
12. Does patient appear ill?	Make patient comfortable	(SDA)

(continued on following page)

3

GENERAL COMPLAINT: EYE DISORDERS *(continued from previous page)*

Disrobing Instructions: None if eye is the only thing involved. Any Sx below neck, disrobe as appropriate.

Vitals: BP & T

Home Care Instructions: If recurring problem and patient has current medicine at home, patient may be instructed to use medicine for 24 hours and follow up with the office. If Sx are mild and have persisted < 24 hrs pt may apply warm compresses. If Sx persist or worsen, pt should notify office ASAP.

Any Modifications: _____

_____

_____

_____

_____

Physician's Approval: _____

GENERAL COMPLAINT: FEVER

COLUMN 1 QUESTIONS (Ask all questions before making any decisions)	COLUMN 2 POSSIBLE PROCEDURES (If patient is in the office)	COLUMN 3 TELEPHONE TRIAGE
1. What is the actual temperature? (list route)		
(pediatric criteria)		
If >101.4° F and < 6 months		(STAT), (SDA)
(Adult criteria)		
If < 103° F and no other Sx present		OTC antipyretic; notify office if Sx worsen.
If >103° F		(SDA)
2. When did fever begin?		
If > 3 days		(SDA)
If < 3 days and below 103° F with no other Sx		OTC antipyretic; information
3. Any history of convulsions?		(STAT)
4. Is patient currently convulsing?	Clear any items from the room that could hurt the patient.	(EMS)
	Never try to confine patient or put anything in patient's mouth.	
5. Does pt have headache?		
If not severe and T < 103° F		Give OTC pain reliever and antipyretic advice
If severe		(STAT)
6. Any neck pain or stiffness?		(STAT)
7. Any other symptoms? (follow questions that go with symptoms, i.e. GI, respiratory, ENT, rash, and urinary Sx)		Follow protocol of related Sx.
8. Does anyone else in the home have similar Sx?		

(continued on following page)

3

GENERAL COMPLAINT: FEVER *(continued from previous page)*

Vitals: BP, T, P & R

Disrobing: Waist Up

Any Modifications:

_____

_____

_____

_____

_____

Physician's Approval: _____

GENERAL COMPLAINT: HEADACHE

COLUMN 1	COLUMN 2	COLUMN 3
QUESTIONS	POSSIBLE PROCEDURES	TELEPHONE TRIAGE
(Ask all questions before making any decisions)	(If patient is in the office)	
1. Exact location of HA and severity (rate pain on a scale from 1-10)	Turn down lights in exam room	
If HA is severe or pain has persisted longer than 24 hours	Turn down lights in exam room	STAT
2. Nausea or vomiting present?	Give patient emesis basin	If other symptoms persist, SDA
3. Recent behavior or personality changes?	Comfort measures	STAT
4. Visual disturbances?	Visual acuity	STAT
5. Drowsiness?	Never leave patient alone	STAT
6. Stiff neck?	Comfort measures	STAT
7. Fever?	Take temperature, comfort measures	If fever has persisted more than 24 hrs or T is > 100° F, SDA; if T is < 100° F or has persisted under 24 hrs give OTC antipyretic information.
8. Has patient had a recent head injury?	Control bleeding (when it applies) Set up suture tray (when it applies)	SDA
Any edema at sight of injury?	Apply ice or cold compresses	Apply ice and SDA
9. Any sinus symptoms?	Possible sinus films	Leading OTC decongestant
If drainage is colored or symptoms are severe:		SDA
10. Does patient have any other medical disorders?		(May be association) SDA

(continued on following page)

GENERAL COMPLAINT: HEADACHE *(continued from previous page)*

COLUMN 1	COLUMN 2	COLUMN 3
QUESTIONS	POSSIBLE PROCEDURES	TELEPHONE TRIAGE
(Ask all questions before making any decisions)	(If patient is in the office)	
11. If HA is mild and has persisted <24 hours and no other Sx persist:	Comfort measures	OTC pain reliever

Vitals: BP & T; if cold Sx are present, include respiration.

Disrobing Instructions: Disrobe as appropriate

Any Modifications: _____

_____

_____

_____

_____

Physician's Approval: _____

GENERAL COMPLAINT: HEAD INJURY

COLUMN 1 QUESTIONS (Ask all questions before making any decisions)	COLUMN 2 POSSIBLE PROCEDURES (If patient is in the office)	COLUMN 3 TELEPHONE TRIAGE
1. When did injury occur?		
2. How did injury occur?		
3. Any bleeding?	Cover with a sterile 4x4, and apply direct pressure and elevate.	Direct pressure and elevation
If bleeding is severe:	Cover with a sterile 4x4, apply direct pressure, elevate, compress nearest pressure point and notify physician ASAP	(EMS)
4. Is wound gaping?	Cover with sterile dressing and set up laceration tray. Follow cleansing procedures for office.	(STAT)
5. Any loss of consciousness?	If patient is unconscious, notify physician at once. Never leave pt unattended.	If unconscious now, (EMS) If conscious now but was unconscious, (STAT)
6. Any mental confusion?	Notify physician ASAP	(STAT)
7. Are pupils unequal, or speech slurred?	Notify physician ASAP	(EMS)
8. Any dizziness?	Never leave pt alone	(STAT)
9. Is pt lethargic?	Notify physician ASAP	(STAT)
10. Any loss of vision?	(Eye tray); possible visual acuity	(STAT)–(ER)
11. Nausea or vomiting?	Provide emesis basin and comfort patient.	(STAT)
12. Severity of pain?	Provide comfort measures (turn down lights) etc.	
If mild, with no other Sx:		OTC analgesic (monitor closely); if Sx do not improve (STAT)
If severe:	Notify physician ASAP	(STAT)

(continued on following page)

GENERAL COMPLAINT: HEAD INJURY *(continued from previous page)*

COLUMN 1	COLUMN 2	COLUMN 3
QUESTIONS	POSSIBLE PROCEDURES	TELEPHONE TRIAGE
(Ask all questions before making any decisions)	(If patient is in the office)	
13. Any discharge coming from nose or mouth? (record what it looks like) blood, clear fluid, etc.?	Notify physician ASAP	(STAT)→(ER)
14. Any neck pain or stiffness since the injury?	Limit the patient's movement; notify physician ASAP	(EMS)
15. Are there any other injuries?	Provide comfort and first aid measures, according to pt's Sx.	If injuries are serious, but not life-threatening (STAT). If injuries are life-threatening (EMS). If injuries are not serious and head injury appears to be minimal, give patient the observation signs listed below. If Sx worsen, pt should notify the office ASAP.
16. Is patient acting normally? If not:		(STAT)

Vitals: BP, P & R

Disrobing Instructions: None, unless other Sx are present as well.

Home Care Management: Observe patient for the following signs: mental confusion, unequal pupils, slurred speech, continuous or excessive vomiting, drainage coming from the ears, nose, or mouth, intensity of headache increases, or patient becomes dizzy. OTC analgesic may be taken to help relieve pain. If patient naps or goes to bed for the evening, the patient should be checked after the first hour of sleep and every 2-3 hours following. Patient should be evaluated for the symptoms listed above. If symptoms are present, the primary physician should be notified right away.

Any Modifications: _____

_____

_____

_____

_____

Physician's Approval: _____

GENERAL COMPLAINT: INSECT STINGS OR BITES

COLUMN 1	COLUMN 2	COLUMN 3
QUESTIONS	POSSIBLE PROCEDURES	TELEPHONE TRIAGE
(Ask all questions before making any decisions)	(If patient is in the office)	
1. Did you see what bit or stung you?		
(If bitten by a centipede, spider, or scorpion): keep insect; bring it to the office		(SDA)
2. Any visible stinger?	Allow physician to see pt. (Do not remove yourself.)	Stinger removal advice
3. Is area around bite swollen, red, or itchy?	Apply ice or cold compress (if no stinger).	If no other Sx present, apply ice and use OTC antihistamine
4. Any difficulty breathing?	Have crash tray or cart and oxygen standing by:	(EMS) ASAP
	Notify physician ASAP (have epinephrine ready)	
5. Swelling around eyes, dizziness, or rash that appears over a large portion of the body?	Notify physician ASAP (have epinephrine ready)	(EMS)
6. Any Hx of severe allergic reactions from previous bites or stings?	Notify physician ASAP (have epinephrine ready)	If Sx present (EMS) ASAP
7. Are Sx getting worse?	Notify physician ASAP (have epinephrine ready)	(EMS) ASAP
8. Does bite look infected?		(SDA)
If insect is a tick:		
1. Is it still embedded in skin?	Set up possible I&D tray	Follow tick removal instructions
2. Does bite look infected?		(SDA)
3. Any rash, fever, headache or muscle aches?		(STAT)
For all types of bites and stings when patient is acting ill:	Notify physician ASAP	(STAT), If Sx are severe, (EMS)

Vitals: BP, T, P & R

Disrobing Instructions: Expose area involved (If rash is present, expose that area as well.) If any respiratory Sx are present, have patient disrobe from waist up.

(continued on following page)

GENERAL COMPLAINT: INSECT STINGS OR BITES *(continued from previous page)*

Stinger Removal Instructions: Should be extracted by scraping stinger off with fingernail or a knife blade. (Never attempt to pull stinger out with fingers or tweezers. This could squeeze more venom into patient. Apply ice to area. Check with physician to see if pt may take OTC antihistamine or apply OTC lotion to area.

Tick Removal Instructions: May cover tick with alcohol or nail polish remover. Grasp the body of the tick firmly with tweezers and remove the head from the skin by using steady pressure. (Never use cigarettes or matches to remove a tick. This could end up burning the patient.)

Any Modifications: _____

_____

_____

_____

_____

Physician's Approval: _____

GENERAL COMPLAINT: LACERATIONS, PUNCTURES, ABRASIONS AND BLEEDING

COLUMN 1	COLUMN 2	COLUMN 3
QUESTIONS	POSSIBLE PROCEDURES	TELEPHONE TRIAGE
(Ask all questions before making any decisions)	(If patient is in the office)	
1. Type of wound and injury	Get cleaning instructions from physician	Cleansing instructions
2. Nature of wound		
3. Is the wound bleeding?	Cover with a sterile 4x4, apply direct pressure, and elevate.	Direct pressure and elevation
If bleeding will not stop:	Compress nearest pressure point and notify physician STAT (set up laceration tray).	(STAT) If patient is hemorrhaging (EMS)
4. Is wound gaping?	Cover with sterile dressing and set up laceration tray.	Cover with sterile dressing (STAT)
5. Any signs of infection, i.e., drainage, red streaks extending from wound, swelling, or general redness?	Do nothing until physician has seen wound	(SDA)
6. Last tetanus shot?	Possible tetanus booster (Never give any injection without a direct order from the physician.)	If patient is behind on tetanus shot (SDA).
7. Any numbness, tingling, or weakness?		(SDA)
Puncture Wound		
1. Any bleeding?		
(Follow instructions for #3 listed above.)		
2. Nature of injury		

(continued on following page)

GENERAL COMPLAINT: LACERATIONS, PUNCTURES, ABRASIONS, AND BLEEDING *(continued from previous page)*

COLUMN 1	COLUMN 2	COLUMN 3
QUESTIONS	POSSIBLE PROCEDURES	TELEPHONE TRIAGE
(Ask all questions before making any decisions)	(If patient is in the office)	
Puncture Wound		
3. Was the puncture object clean or dirty (rusty)?	Get cleaning instructions from physician	If minor, follow cleaning instructions found at the bottom of chart.
4. Last tetanus shot?	Possible tetanus shot	If patient is behind on tetanus shot (SDA).
5. Any signs of infection?		
(Follow instructions for #5 on the previous page)		
6. Is wound very deep?	Set up for possible suture tray	If yes (SDA)
7. Any foreign material visible?	Set up I&D Tray	(SDA)
Abrasions		

Abrasions can usually be handled at home. Follow cleaning instructions listed on the next page. Abrasions are very susceptible to infection. If there are any signs of infection, notify the office immediately.

Home care cleaning instructions for lacerations, abrasions, and punctures: Flush wound with cool water. Scrub gently with soap and water and rinse. Apply antiseptic, i.e., hydrogen peroxide, antibiotic ointment, etc. Cover with bandage or sterile dressing. Notify office if any signs of infection.

Vitals: BP, T & P

Disrobing Instructions: Expose area or areas involved.

Any Modifications: _____

_____

_____

_____

_____

Physician's Approval: _____

GENERAL COMPLAINT: RASHES AND SKIN DISORDERS

COLUMN 1	COLUMN 2	COLUMN 3
QUESTIONS	POSSIBLE PROCEDURES	TELEPHONE TRIAGE
(Ask all questions before making any decisions)	(If patient is in the office)	
1. Description of rash and location	Special light (black light), magnifying glass, etc.	
If rash is combined with any of the following: fever, sore throat, or earache	Possible throat culture if sore throat is present.	
When rash is unidentifiable:		(SDA)
2. Has patient started any new medications recently?	Have list of all medications currently being taken by patient.	(SDA) Patient may be having an allergic reaction to the medication (should be checked).
3. Any change in laundry detergents or fabric softeners? Any new clothing or worn another's clothing?		Patient should be advised to stop using the items that could be causing the rash. OTC antihistamine. If there is no change in a 24-hr period, patient is to notify office.
4. Has patient been exposed to any new chemicals?		(SDA)
Chicken Pox		
1. When was patient exposed?		
2. Any URI symptoms present?		
If severe:		(SDA)
3. Any convulsions, severe pain, especially head pain, or stiff neck present?	If convulsing, clear the area. Have someone notify physician ASAP.	(STAT) (EMS), if convulsing
4. Is patient lethargic?		(STAT)
5. Do pox look infected?		(SDA)
6. Location of pox. If located on eyes:		(SDA)

(continued on following page)

GENERAL COMPLAINT: RASHES AND SKIN DISORDERS *(continued from previous page)*

COLUMN 1	COLUMN 2	COLUMN 3
QUESTIONS (Ask all questions before making any decisions)	POSSIBLE PROCEDURES (If patient is in the office)	TELEPHONE TRIAGE
Chicken Pox		
7. If mother is certain of the diagnosis, and no complications exist:	Home care instructions, listed below.	
Poison Ivy		
1. If infected or any swelling:		(SDA)
2. Location, if on face or genitals:		(SDA)
3. If no complications exist:		Home care instructions, listed below.
Acne		
1. All patients with acne should be seen initially by physician for treatment plan:		(WK)
Moles, Skin Tags, and Warts		
Patients will normally want these removed.	Set up excision tray, Hyfrecator equipment, liquid nitrogen, etc.	(WK)
List location, length of time, present changes.	Have biopsy containers available.	If patient is apprehensive, (24)
Scabies	Set up slide and blade	(SDA)–(24)

Vitals: Usually not necessary, unless it is the standard routine of the office.

Disrobing Instructions: Expose area involved.

Chicken Pox Home Care Management: Cut nails to avoid possible scratches, tub bath with Aveeno oatmeal bath or Alpha Keri lotion (follow instructions on package insert). For itching, give OTC antihistamine information; pain and fever give OTC pain and fever relief information.

Poison Ivy Home Care Management: Apply calamine lotion with cotton ball. OTC antihistamine information for itching; OTC pain reliever for pain.

(continued on following page)

GENERAL COMPLAINT: RASHES AND SKIN DISORDERS *(continued from previous page)*

Any Modifications:

_____

_____

_____

_____

_____

Physician's Approval:_____

GENERAL COMPLAINT: STOMACH PAIN, NAUSEA, VOMITING, AND DIARRHEA

COLUMN 1 QUESTIONS (Ask all questions before making any decisions)	COLUMN 2 POSSIBLE PROCEDURES (If patient is in the office)	COLUMN 3 TELEPHONE TRIAGE
1. Location and intensity of pain (scale-1-10)		
2. Last BM and texture (if abnormal)	Possible rectal exam/stool cultures	(24)-(48)
3. Any diarrhea?		
If > than 5-6 watery stools in a 12-hour period	Possible rectal exam/stool cultures	SDA
If amount is < 5-6 stools in a 12 or less hour time frame:	Possible rectal exam/stool cultures As Sx subside, pt may start on Brat diet (listed below).	Clear liquid diet for 24 hours (listed below).
4. Nausea or vomiting	Give patient emesis basin	
If patient appears to be dehydrated or Sx are in conjunction with severe pain:	Wait for physician's instructions	STAT (especially infants, as they can dehydrate in a short amount of time)
If Sx are mild:		Give pt rehydration instructions, listed below. Give patient dehydration signs, listed below.
5. Is blood present in stool?	Possible rectal exam/stool culture	SDA
6. Is mucus or pus in stool?	Possible rectal exam/stool culture	SDA
7. Fever (if over 101° F and pain is intense):		SDA
8. Any belching or flatus?		
9. Does patient have a Hx of stomach problems?		SDA
10. Has patient traveled recently, tried new foods, or does anyone else in the family have Sx?		If patient has traveled abroad recently, has stomach cramping, N/V, or diarrhea, SDA.
11. If no other Sx other than pain and the pain is intense:	Provide comfort measures for patient	SDA
mild and intermittent:	Provide comfort measures for patient	OTC antacid, F/U with office if Sx worsen

(continued on following page)

GENERAL COMPLAINT: STOMACH PAIN, NAUSEA, VOMITING, AND DIARRHEA *(continued from previous page)*

Vitals: BP & T

Disrobing Instructions: Fully

Clear Liquid Diet: For the first 24 hrs patient should only take in clear liquids, i.e., flat sodas, weak tea, and gelatin. Can offer Pedialyte to infants. Liquids should be offered approximately every 2 hrs. Patient should then follow Brat diet.

BRAT DIET: Pt can start adding bananas, rice, applesauce, and toast to diet for approx. 24-48 hours. Normal diet may be resumed once diarrhea has stopped.

Dehydration Signs: Listlessness, dry mouth, sunken eyeballs, no urine in last 8-10 hours or urine is very dark in color and has a strong odor.

Rehydration Instructions: Offer fluids as often as possible, encourage patient to drink fluids like Gatorade in adults and Pedialyte in infants. If Sx persist > than _____ hours, patient should notify office ASAP.

Any Modifications: _____

_____

_____

_____

_____

Physician's Approval: _____

GENERAL COMPLAINT: STRAINS, SPRAINS, AND FRACTURES

COLUMN 1	COLUMN 2	COLUMN 3
QUESTIONS	POSSIBLE PROCEDURES	TELEPHONE TRIAGE
(Ask all questions before making any decisions)	(If patient is in the office)	
1. What part of the body was injured?		
2. When and how did injury occur? (be specific)		
3. Any swelling	Elevate and apply ice pack, possible Xray	Elevate, apply ice, (SDA)
4. Does pain intensify with movement?	Elevate, possible Xrays	(STAT)
Is pain severe?	Elevate, possible Xrays	(STAT)
5. Is area red, swollen, or warm?	Keep extremity elevated	(SDA)
6. Is skin broken?	Possible laceration tray, tetanus shot	If gapping (STAT)
If bone is protruding through the skin:	Cover area with sterile drape; notify physician ASAP and treat pt for shock.	(EMS)
7. Any fever?		(SDA)
8. Does patient appear ill?	Provide comfort measures	(SDA)

STRAINS

Strains are usually the result of overworking a muscle. If patient can trace back to a new sport or new form of exercise and there are no signs of anything more serious going on, such as a sprain or fracture, then home care management advice may be an option.

Home Care Management Advice for Minor Strained Muscles: Rest, OTC analgesic information. Apply ice 3-4 times a day for 15-20 minutes until Sx improve. Call office if symptoms worsen or if pain persists for more than 3 days.

Possible fractures and sprains should always be seen initially.

Vitals: BP & T _____

Any Modifications: _____

_____

Physician's Approval: _____

GENERAL COMPLAINT: URINARY SYMPTOMS

COLUMN 1	COLUMN 2	COLUMN 3
QUESTIONS	POSSIBLE PROCEDURES	TELEPHONE TRIAGE
(Ask all questions before making any decisions)	(If patient is in the office)	
1. Burning or pain upon urination?	Possible UA and C&S	(SDA)-(24)
2. Urinary frequency or nocturia?	Possible UA and C&S	(SDA)-(24)
3. Fever (record T and route)?		If > 100° F (SDA)
4. Any back pain or pressure?	Possible UA and C&S, possible Xray	If other Sx present, (SDA)
5. Any abdominal pain or pressure?	Possible pelvic exam, if female; rectal exam in male	If other Sx present, (SDA)
6. Any nausea or vomiting?	Give patient emesis basin	If severe, (SDA)
7. Any Hx of UTIs?		
8. Pus or blood present in urine?	Possible UA and C&S, if blood is present	(SDA)
	Possible Xray	
9. (Female) Any vaginal symptoms?	Possible pelvic tray, STD cultures	(SDA)
(LMP)	Possible pregnancy test	If period > 2 weeks late, (SDA)-(24)
10. (Male) Any penile symptoms?	Possible STD cultures	(SDA)
11. (Female) Itching of rectum?	Possible rectal exam (anoscope)	(SDA)

Vitals: BP & T

Disrobing Instructions: If symptoms are minor, none. If symptoms involve genital area, waist down.

If abdominal or back pain or pressure is present, waist up. Females may leave bra on.

Any Modifications:

Physician's Approval:

GENERAL COMPLAINT: VAGINAL OR PENILE SYMPTOMS

COLUMN 1 QUESTIONS (Ask all questions before making any decisions)	COLUMN 2 POSSIBLE PROCEDURES (If patient is in the office)	COLUMN 3 TELEPHONE TRIAGE
1. Any vaginal or penile discharge?	Possible pelvic exam (female), STD cultures, (both male and female)	If no other Sx present (24)-(48)
(List color and odor, if unusual)	Possible urethral exam (male)	If other Sx present, (SDA)
2. Any vaginal itching (female)?	Set up for pelvic exam (hanging drop, wet prep)	If no other Sx give OTC vaginal cream information. (Pt should F/U with office) Contact office if Sx worsen.
3. Any penile itching (male)?	Possible urethral exam	(24)-(48)
4. Any urinary Sx?	Possible UA and C&S	(SDA)-(24)
5. Any abdominal pain or pressure?		If severe, (SDA)
		If in conjunction with other Sx, (SDA)
6. Any lower back pain or pressure?	Possible UA and C&S	(SDA)-(24)
7. If female, list LMP. Is it normal?		
If > than 10 days late:	Possible pregnancy test	(SDA)-(24)
8. Pain during intercourse?	Possible pelvic exam (female), (STD culture)	If combined with other Sx, SDA. If not (24)-(48).
9. Number of sexual partners?		
If STD is suspected:	Possible pelvic exam (female), (STD culture)	When combined with other Sx, (SDA)-(24).
10. Fever?		

Vitals: BP & T

Disrobing Instructions: Waist down if Sx stay below waist. Completely if Sx move above waist.

STD Cultures: Gonorrhea and chlamydia cultures most common.

(continued on following page)

GENERAL COMPLAINT: VAGINAL OR PENILE SYMPTOMS *(continued from previous page)*

Other Testing: (KOH, Wet Mount) If discharge is white, resembles cottage cheese, smells like baking bread, and involves vaginal itching, redness, or burning, set up for a wet mount and KOH testing. If in office, place swabbed contents into 1/2 cc of saline. Roll swab onto slide and add 1 drop of 10% KOH. Apply coverslip and read. If patient's symptoms are a frothy grayish yellow discharge with a fishy odor, set up wet mount only.

Any Modifications:

Physician's Approval: _____

SECTION

4

OBSTETRICS AND GYNECOLOGY

Introduction

The Obstetrics and Gynecology (OB/GYN) section deals with common diseases and disorders that arise in an OB/GYN setting.

This section will provide the assistant with better assessment skills in the OB/GYN office as well as with general anticipation skills.

There are eight divisions in this section. Half of the contents is geared toward the GYN patient, and the other half deals with the OB patient.

The divisions are as follows:

1. Annual Pap and Pelvic Exam

2. Common Gynecological Disorders

3. Female Vaginal Disorders (Vaginitis)

4. Female Reproductive Diseases and Disorders

5. Gynecological Diagnostic Tests and Procedures

6. Routine Prenatal Exam

7. Obstetrical Diseases and Disorders

8. Obstetrical Diagnostic Tests and Procedures

This section will be beneficial to the student in the classroom as well as the veteran assistant who is already working in the field.

It is important that the assistant take the time to review the charts with the physician prior to implementing them into the practice. Any necessary adjustments should be made before the physician signs off the chart that pertains to your facility's needs.

GENERAL COMPLAINT: ANNUAL PAP AND PELVIC EXAM

QUESTIONS	SPECIAL EQUIPMENT, SUPPLIES, OR PROCEDURES
1. Last pap test and results	
2. Any current vaginal Sx?	Set up appropriate cultures
3. Form of birth control?	
4. G (Gravida)	
5. T (Term Parity)	
6. P (Preterm Parity)	
7. A (Abortions) Elective or spontaneous?	
8. L (Living Children)	
9. List any gynecological surgeries	
10. Number of sexual partners? (Physician may want to ask this question.)	
11. Any pain during intercourse?	
12. Any other Sx present?	
13. Any urinary Sx?	Possible UA and C&S
14. LMP	If >10 days late for menses, possible pregnancy test.

Vitals: WT, HT, BP

Tray Set Ups and Cultures: Pap tray. Some physicians will routinely want GC and chlamydia cultures set up, while other offices will only want those cultures if the patient has vaginal Sx. (Pap tray set up can be found in Section 8 in the tray set ups.)

Other Procedures and Cultures: Wet prep (Hanging drop), done when the doctor suspects the patient has trichomoniasis or gardnerella infections. Set up test tube with 0.5 ml of saline. Place specimen in test tube. Take specimen and spread over slide. Reinsert applicator as many times as it takes to get a drop large enough to cover with coverslip. Place under microscope, high power. KOH, the same procedure as wet prep, but place a drop of KOH on slide before putting coverslip on slide. GC culture, modified thayer martin culture, chlamydia culture. Must be stored in chlamydia culture transport vial.

(continued on following page)

GENERAL COMPLAINT: ANNUAL PAP AND PELVIC EXAM *(continued from previous page)*

Codes and Abbreviations: Sx-Symptoms, UA-Urinalysis, C&S-Culture and Sensitivity, WT-Weight, HT-Height, BP-Blood Pressure, T-Temperature, Gravida-Number of pregnancies, Term Parity-Number of deliveries at term (38-42 weeks' gestation), Preterm Parity-Number of preterm deliveries, Abortions-Termination of birth prior to 24 weeks' gestation. May be spontaneous, therapeutic, or induced. Living children-# of living children at this time.

Any Modifications:

_____

_____

_____

_____

Physician's Approval: _____

COMMON GYNECOLOGICAL DISORDERS

PREMENSTRUAL SYNDROME (PMS)

Definition	Cause	Symptoms	Treatment
A term used to describe a group of physical or behavioral changes that some women experience prior to the onset of menses each month.	Not certain what causes PMS. Could be related to the change in hormone levels that occurs before menses each month.	**Physical Changes:** Bloating, weight gain, abdominal swelling, swollen hands and feet, headache, clumsiness, constipation, fatigue, and breast soreness. **Behavioral Changes:** Depression, mood swings, inability to concentrate, changes in sex drive, anxiety, and tension.	No cure, but individual symptoms can be relieved through medications. Examples include diuretics, oral contraceptives, vitamins, and natural progesterone. Prozac and exercise have also proven to be beneficial in the treatment of PMS in many women. **Diet Suggestions:** Reducing the amount of salt and caffeine intake prior to menses will help eliminate some of the common symptoms that occur with PMS. Examples of foods that contain caffeine include coffee, tea, colas, and chocolate.

ENDOMETRIOSIS

Definition	Cause	Symptoms	Treatment
Endometrial tissue grows outside of the uterus, including the ovaries, fallopian tubes, bladder, ligaments, vagina, and bowel.	Exact cause unknown; one theory is referred to as retrograde menstruation.	Patient may be asymptomatic, while others might experience light to severe pain before and during menses, irregular or heavy periods, and pain during intercourse. In severe cases, the patient may have a hard time conceiving.	Surgical treatment and drug therapy. Some drug options include oral contraceptives, male hormones, and progesterones. Lupron injections also work well. Conservative surgical treatment means the physician would only remove individual areas of tissue containing the endometriosis. Nonconservative methods include a partial or total hysterectomy.

UTERINE FIBROIDS

Definition	Cause	Symptoms	Treatment
Round growths of muscle tissue found in the walls of the uterus. Usually benign and harmless. They can start out the size of a pea but grow rapidly throughout a woman's reproductive years.	Not certain. They do tend to be hereditary, however.	May be none. Patient might have abnormal uterine bleeding, back pain, or difficulty getting pregnant. Achiness, heaviness, and fullness also are symptoms.	Monitoring the fibroids. Removal of the fibroids, a hysterectomy, and in some cases endometrial ablation is an alternative. Lupron injections help to shrink leiomyomas.

FACTS: In some cases, uterine fibroids have been known to become cancerous. Constant monitoring is a must.

4

FEMALE VAGINAL DISORDERS

VAGINITIS

CANDIDA, MONILIASIS (YEAST)

SYMPTOMS	DIAGNOSTIC TOOLS	TREATMENT	INTERCOURSE
Scanty white discharge that resembles cottage cheese. Odor: None, or smells like baking bread. Vaginal redness and burning. Severe itching. Intercourse may be painful.	**(IO):** Place swabbed contents into 1/2 cc of saline. Roll swab onto slide and add 1 drop of 10% KOH. Apply coverslip and read. **(SO):** Place in appropriate transport medium, e.g., culturette	Antifungal creams or suppositories, i.e., Nystatin, (Mycostatin); Monistat, (Miconazole); Gyn-Lotrimin, (Clotrimazole) Oral Diflucan (1 time dose works well.)	Should avoid until asymptomatic or have partner wear condom until asymptomatic.

Possible contributors or causes: pregnancy, birth control pills, diabetes, antibiotics, and sometimes sexual intercourse

TRICHOMONIASIS (CAUSED BY THE PARASITE *TRICHOMONAS VAGINALIS*)

SYMPTOMS	DIAGNOSTIC TOOLS	TREATMENT	INTERCOURSE
Thin, frothy vaginal discharge. Color: Usually greyish-yellow; Odor: Fishy odor, may have urinary symptoms. "Trich" often invades the urinary tract, causing symptoms. Painful intercourse also may be a symptom.	**(IO):** Set up wet mount, Place swab with specimen into 1/2 cc of saline. Roll swab onto slide and apply coverslip. Put under microscope to read. **(SO):** Place in sterile culture tube that contains saline, like the culturette.	Oral medication, e.g., Flagyl, (metronidazole) Metrogel (vaginal gel)	Okay if both the patient and partner are treated at the same time, otherwise patient should wait until infection is gone.

Possible contributors or causes: sexual intercourse (not necessary though), shared towels, sitting on toilet seats.

IMPORTANT: Both the patient and the patient's partner must be treated, or the risk of reinfection occurs.

GARDNERELLA (*GARDNERELLA VAGINALIS*)

SYMPTOMS	DIAGNOSTIC TOOLS	TREATMENT	INTERCOURSE
Watery whitish or greyish vaginal discharge. Odor: Offensive odor produced by the bacteria. Usually no itching or burning sensation unless infection is acute.	**(IO):** Set up wet mount, (directions listed above.) Look for clue cells. **(IO):** Set up Wiff Test. Physician will place a few drops of KOH onto the speculum to detect a fishy odor. **(SO):** Sterile culture tube, like the culturette.	Oral antibiotics; Metronidazole or Flagyl 500 mg. po, bid × 5 days.	Okay if both patient and partner are being treated at the same time, otherwise patient should wait until asymptomatic.

(continued on following page)

FEMALE VAGINAL DISORDERS *(continued from previous page)*

GARDNERELLA (*GARDNERELLA VAGINALIS*)

Possible contributors or causes: Can be transmitted sexually and also can exist in small amounts in the vagina without causing symptoms. Once the pH level decreases, the hemophilus can grow in large quantities, causing infection. Can cause premature rupture of membranes while pregnant. Both the patient and partner must be treated to avoid reinfection.

WAYS TO AVOID GETTING VAGINITIS

1. Wear cotton underwear. (The cotton will allow the air to circulate better.)
2. Always wipe from front to back. (Use white tissue only.)
3. Avoid douching without a physician's approval.
4. Avoid wearing tight-fitting jeans or pants.
5. Alert doctor that you are prone to vaginitis when taking antibiotics. (Watch for symptoms.)
6. Avoid using deodorant sprays. (These have chemicals that can irritate the vulva.)
7. Wash vulva area and perineum daily. Use unscented soaps and nondeodorant soaps whenever possible.
8. Change out of wet suit into dry clothes right away.

Abbreviations: IO means: If the specimen is tested in the office you may want to do the following:

SO means: If the specimen is sent out of the office, you may want to do the following:

FEMALE REPRODUCTIVE DISEASES AND DISORDERS

VENEREAL DISEASE

GONORRHEA

SYMPTOMS	DIAGNOSTIC TOOLS	TREATMENT	INTERCOURSE
Initially, a yellowish purulent vaginal discharge. Urinary discomfort and frequency also may be present. Progressive symptoms may include acute abdominal pain and fever (PID symptoms).	**(IO)** or **(SO):** Specimen should be plated on an enriched medium known as chocolate agar. Thayer Martin is a good example. These agar plates should be stored in the refrigerator but brought to room temperature before plating. Needs a high CO_2 environment. Follow directions for method used. (May do a gram stain.)	Rocephin (Ceftriaxone) IM, followed up with an oral dose of Vibramycin (Doxycycline).	Must be avoided until physician gives patient a clean bill of health. All partners must be treated.

CHLAMYDIA

SYMPTOMS	DIAGNOSTIC TOOLS	TREATMENT	INTERCOURSE
Many patients will be asymptomatic. If symptoms are present, they will include a thick white-yellow discharge, odor, usually negative, and in advanced cases, acute abdominal pain and fever may exist. (PID symptoms)	**(IO):** Usually sent out. May do a gram stain. **(SO):** Cell culture isolation. May draw blood for Serum-Antibody Detection or Direct-Antigen Detection.	Usually Tetracycline (Achromycin Ophthalmic), or Vibramycin (Doxycycline)	Must be avoided until physician gives patient a clean bill of health. All partners must be treated.

HERPES SIMPLEX, TYPE II

SYMPTOMS	DIAGNOSTIC TOOLS	TREATMENT	INTERCOURSE
Initially: Painful blisters in vagina, cervix, and vulva. Initial episode may last from 10 days to 2 weeks, followed by flu-like symptoms. Virus will stay in the body forever. Outbreaks may recur throughout the patient's lifetime.	**(IO):** Usually sent out. Physician may perform Tzanck Smear; will look at the cells taken from sores. **(SO):** Herpes Culture (Viral Media) or Serology Tests can be done to measure increases in antibody production against the herpes virus.	Zovirax (Acyclovir) if given early enough, can reduce the severity and length of the outbreak. No cure. Will suggest various treatments and medications to alleviate symptoms. See following page for helpful hints.	None during outbreaks

(continued on following page)

FEMALE REPRODUCTIVE DISEASES AND DISORDERS *(continued from previous page)*

HELPFUL HINTS TO THINK ABOUT DURING HERPES OUTBREAKS:

1. Keep sores dry (blow drying sores on low heat may help speed healing).
2. Take OTC analgesics to combat pain.
3. Avoid using topical ointments.
4. Avoid picking at the sores.
5. Wash sores with soap and water.
6. Avoid wearing tight clothes (they trap moisture).
7. Avoid touching eyes (virus could be in fingertips).
8. Do not share linens when sores are present.

IMPORTANT POINTS ABOUT HERPES: Patient must fight to keep up immunity. Get plenty of rest and eat properly. Avoid stress as much as possible, as this will wear down your body's natural immunity.

SYPHILIS (SYPH)

SYMPTOMS	DIAGNOSTIC TOOLS	TREATMENT	INTERCOURSE
Initially chancre sore on vulva, vagina, cervix, in the mouth, anus, or lips. A rash may appear for a short time following the chancre. The spirochete can live in the body for years, destroying additional tissue.	**(IO):** Usually sent out. **(SO):** RPR, VDRL	Penicillin or other antibiotics	None until treatment is concluded and patient is asymptomatic.

CONDYLOMA (GENITAL WARTS) HPV, (HUMAN PAPILLOMA VIRUS)

SYMPTOMS	DIAGNOSTIC TOOLS	TREATMENT	INTERCOURSE
Can look like tiny warts, bumps, or cauliflower growths; granules may be flat and barely visible. Color: Flesh-colored, pink, or darker than surrounding tissue.	**(IO):** Pelvic exam (visual examination) **(IO):** Colposcopy (visual examination) **(SO):** Pap test	Pedophyllin (topical chemical) should not be administered during pregnancy. TCA (topical chemical) may be administered during pregnancy. 5-Fluorouracil, a cream that is used for warts inside the urethra. Heat, laser, and freezing are other effective methods to eliminate warts.	Stop for a brief time after treatment. This helps the overall healing process. Partner should be treated to prevent reinfection.

The main concern with patients who are infected with herpes and undiagnosed or untreated condyloma is the increased risk of genital or cervical cancer. Seek immediate attention and follow up regularly.

(continued on following page)

4

FEMALE REPRODUCTIVE DISEASES AND DISORDERS *(continued from previous page)*

AIDS (ACQUIRED IMMUNODEFICIENCY SYNDROME), RESULT OF BEING HIV-POSITIVE

SYMPTOMS	DIAGNOSTIC TOOLS	TREATMENT	INTERCOURSE
Enlargement of lymph nodes, persistent diarrhea, repeated fevers and night sweats, chronic fatigue, anorexia, pharyngitis, arthralgia, and adenopathy. In progressed cases: dementia, memory loss, nervous disorders, and multiple purplish dark red blotches may be found on the head, trunk, neck and arms as a result of a neoplasm called Kaposi's Sarcoma. Other internal organs also may be involved. Once patient has progressed to symptoms of AIDS, death is imminent.	Diagnosis of HIV: Elisa Test (repeat if positive); if still positive, Western Blot is done to confirm diagnosis. Diagnosis of AIDS: The presence of AIDS-related disorders and a T-Cell count of 200 or less.	No Cure: ZDU, Zidovudine, formally known as AZT, and other drugs are used to stimulate immunity and alleviate various symptoms.	Should be avoided. If this is not possible extreme caution should be taken. The use of condoms cannot be over-emphasized.

PELVIC INFLAMMATORY DISEASE

SYMPTOMS	DIAGNOSTIC TOOLS	TREATMENT	INTERCOURSE
Severe lower abdominal pain or tenderness, purulent cervical discharge, fever and adjacent tenderness also may be present. More common in young girls in their late teens and early 20s who are sexually active, but seen in other age groups as well.	**(SO):** Set up GC and chlamydia culture. **(IO):** Set up for a gram stain. Physician may want to do a CBC and ESR. May also need to schedule a laparoscopy to confirm diagnosis. Proper lighting for visual examination.	Immediate intervention is important because of the risk of sterility. Antibiotics such as Cefoxitin 2 g, IM, followed by Probenicid, 1 g, orally. Patient should follow up with doxycycline 100 mg, bid x 10 days. In advanced cases, patients should be hospitalized with IV antibiotics.	Should not have intercourse until patient has completed treatment and has gotten physician's okay.

Abbreviations: IO means the specimen is tested in the office; SO means it is sent out of the office.

GYNECOLOGICAL DIAGNOSTIC TESTS AND PROCEDURES

TEST NAME	DESCRIPTION	INDICATED CONDITIONS
COLPOSCOPY	Examination of the vaginal and cervical tissues using an instrument called a colposcope.	Abnormal Pap smears. Used to select sites of abnormal tissue growth for biopsy and to evaluate benign lesions and define tumor extension.
LEEP PROCEDURE	Loop Electrosurgical Excision Procedure (LEEP) quickly removes abnormal tissue from the cervix without destroying it, so further examination may be done to ensure that no cancer is present.	Dysplasia
HYSTEROSCOPY	A hysteroscope is inserted into the uterus to permit visual examination of the uterus and its surrounding tissue.	Uterine fibroids, bleeding, and other abnormalities. Abnormal tissue, tumors, and fibroids may be extracted for biopsy purposes.
PAP SMEAR	Tissue is extracted from the vagina and cervix and sent to a laboratory for analysis.	Prevention tool for vaginal, cervical and uterine cancer.
ENDOMETRIAL BIOPSY	Removing tissue from the uterine endometrium for evaluative purposes.	Same as hysteroscopy
LAPAROSCOPY/PELVISCOPY	Abdominal exploration through an instrument called a laparoscope. This procedure allows the physician to view the uterus, fallopian tubes, and ovaries through one tiny incision. The removal of fibroids may be performed using this method.	Adhesions, fibroids, cysts, endometriosis, and ectopic pregnancies. Routine gynecological procedures like tubal sterilization and hysterectomies are performed using this procedure.
ULTRASONOGRAPHY	Harmless soundwaves instead of Xrays to produce images of the uterus and ovaries.	Used to determine fetal age, size, and various fetal abnormalities. Also used to detect abnormalities and growths of the ovaries and uterus, including tubal pregnancies.

4

(continued on following page)

GYNECOLOGICAL DIAGNOSTIC TESTS AND PROCEDURES *(continued from previous page)*

TEST NAME	DESCRIPTION	INDICATED CONDITIONS
DILATION AND CURETTAGE	Dilating the cervix and scraping off some of the endometrial lining.	Heavy bleeding, possible miscarriages, and also can be used to remove small growths. It also can provide biopsy samples for evaluation.
ENDOMETRIAL ABLATION	The use of an electric current or a laser to destroy the entire uterine lining.	Its use may be indicated to control heavy bleeding. Should not be used in patients who might want to become pregnant in the future because pregnancy and childbirth are no longer possible after this procedure.
SALPINGOGRAPHY	Radiographic study of the fallopian tubes into which a radiopaque dye is introduced to check tube patency.	Performed on women who are having a hard time conceiving.

ROUTINE PRENATAL EXAM

GENERAL QUESTIONS	SPECIAL EQUIPMENT, SUPPLIES, OR PROCEDURES	TELEPHONE TRIAGE
EDC (Expected Date of Confinement) (Ask for LMP on first visit)	Fetal monitor, ultrasonic gel and tape measure	If new patient who wants to confirm that she is pregnant and is at least 7-10 days late, set up an appointment for a pregnancy test.
Any swelling in hands, feet, or face? (Is it pitting edema?)	Have patient lie on left side, and keep feet elevated.	If there is a great deal of swelling or the patient has pitting edema, try to set a same-day appointment.
Any vaginal bleeding? List amount if possible, i.e., teaspoon, tablespoon, etc. List actual color of blood. Has patient passed any clots or other strange tissue? Any cramping?	Set up for pelvic exam.	If bleeding is heavy or bright red, send patient to hospital for further evaluation. If patient has passed any blood clots or tissue, instruct pt to put the clot or tissue into a container and go to the hospital. If patient has very little bleeding and it is a dark-brown color, have patient stop activity and lie down with feet elevated. Notify office right away if bleeding changes in amount or color, or if pain is present.
(As patients get closer to their due date, there is the possibility of an amniotic leak. If patient states that she is leaking a clear vaginal fluid, i.e., like urine, record how much she has lost, what time it started, and the color of the fluid.)	Set up test kit.	If patient feels certain of amniotic leak, send to labor and delivery. If uncertain and leak appears to be small, set up an appointment ASAP.
Any unusual vaginal discharge? (List color and amount.)	Set up for possible pelvic exam.	Set up an appointment within the following 24-48 hours, if patient is concerned.
Any headaches, dizziness, or vision problems?		If severe, set up an appointment for the same day. If mild, suggest possible comfort measures approved by the physician.

(continued on following page)

4

ROUTINE PRENATAL EXAM *(continued from previous page)*

GENERAL QUESTIONS	SPECIAL EQUIPMENT, SUPPLIES, OR PROCEDURES	TELEPHONE TRIAGE
Any nausea or vomiting?	Give emesis basin and make the patient comfortable.	If severe, check to see if the physician wants the patient to go to the hospital or come into the office. If slight, provide patient with home treatment measures.
Appetite		
DISROBING PROCEDURES:	FIRST EXAM: Fully disrobe; SUBSEQUENT VISITS: Tummy exposed, week 36-40, waist down (will vary with the physician)	
ROUTINE PROCEDURES:	FIRST EXAM: Prenatal profile, (consists of various lab work); Pap test, GC culture, chlamydia cultures, UA, weight, blood pressure, detailed health history and nutrition counseling.	
	SUBSEQUENT VISITS: Weight check, blood pressure, UA dipstick (protein and glucose).	
	VARIOUS INTERVAL EXAMS: Alpha-1 Fetoprotein (15-20 weeks), GTT (24-28 weeks), amniocentesis (no earlier than 14 weeks' gestation), Rhogam (28 weeks).	

Any Modifications: _____

_____

_____

_____

_____

Physician's Approval: _____

OBSTETRICAL DISEASES AND DISORDERS

PREECLAMPSIA/ECLAMPSIA, PIH, OR TOXEMIA

Definition	Symptoms	Diagnostic Tools	Treatment
Mild Preeclampsia—the development of albuminuria, hypertension, or edema between 20 weeks' gestation and the first week of postpartum.	Pt develops a BP > 140/90 or a BP which increases more than 30 mm/Hg systolic or increases more than 15 mm/Hg diastolic.	BP check, UA dipstick for protein, CBC, UA, BUN, creatinine and electrolytes. Platelets and a 24-hour urine also may be performed.	Pt should be placed on bed rest and instructed to lie on her L side. Pt should be advised to increase water intake. If Sx worsen or condition advances to severe preeclampsia, the patient should be placed in the hospital on IV. Delivery is performed as soon as it is safe for both the mother and baby. If the mother's condition worsens, the physician may need to deliver, even if it is dangerous to the fetus.
Eclampsia—the development of coma or convulsive seizures.	Patient usually develops coma or convulsive seizures.	Observation and same as above.	Same as advanced preeclampsia.

HYDATIFORM MOLE

Definition	Symptoms	Diagnostic Tools	Treatment
The end stage of a degenerating pregnancy in which the villi will swell and the trophoblastic elements will proliferate. May be benign but in some cases is malignant.	Rapid increase in the size of the uterus. It is much larger than it should be by date. Possible vaginal bleeding, lack of fetal movement, severe nausea and vomiting. Passage of tissue that looks like grapes will sometimes occur.	HCG levels are usually elevated; ultrasonography is usually done.	Removal of the mole, D&C, sometimes a hysterectomy. Treatment will depend on the individual case.

PLACENTA PREVIA

Definition	Symptoms	Diagnostic Tools	Treatment
Implantation of the placenta near or over the cervix.	Severe bleeding during the last half of the pregnancy.	Ultrasound and vaginal examination	Bed rest and hospitalization, probable C-section at the time of birth.

(continued on following page)

4

OBSTETRICAL DISEASES AND DISORDERS *(continued from previous page)*

ABRUPTIO PLACENTAE

Definition	Symptoms	Diagnostic Tools	Treatment
Premature separation of the placenta from the uterus.	Possible vaginal bleeding, a tender or contracted uterus, fetal distress or death, and maternal shock, in some cases.	Ultrasound and vaginal examination	Bed rest, hospitalization, delivery (possible C-section or vaginal delivery, depending on the particular case)

MALPRESENTATION

Definition	Symptoms	Diagnostic Tools	Treatment
This is a condition in which the baby is not headfirst. The baby may be in a transverse position.	None	Physical assessment and ultrasound	At the time of birth, the physician may need to consider forcep delivery or C-section.

PREMATURE LABOR AND DELIVERY

Definition	Symptoms	Diagnostic Tools	Treatment
Defined as labor that begins before the 37th week of pregnancy.	Menstrual-like cramps, pelvic pressure, light bleeding, low back pain, vaginal discharge, and diarrhea.	Physical examination	Medications to stop the labor

PREMATURE RUPTURE OF THE MEMBRANES

Definition	Symptoms	Diagnostic Tools	Treatment
Rupture of the amniotic fluid sac prior to the onset of labor.	Clear or milky fluid coming from the vagina.	pH kit	Bed rest at home or in the hospital to help reduce the risk of infection. If patient is far enough along, labor is sometimes induced.

(continued on following page)

OBSTETRICAL DISEASES AND DISORDERS *(continued from previous page)*

LABOR DISORDERS

Definition	Symptoms	Diagnostic Tools	Treatment
Any deviation in the progress of labor. This can include deviations in contractions, dilatation, or passage of the fetus through the birth canal.	Patient usually does not progress the way she should.	Fetal and maternal monitoring; physical assessment	Inducing labor with a drug like Pitocin; in some cases, an emergency C-section is recommended.

GESTATIONAL DIABETES OR GLUCOSE INTOLERANCE

Definition	Symptoms	Diagnostic Tools	Treatment
An increase in blood sugar during pregnancy.	Polydipsia, polyuria, polyphagia, a larger-than-normal baby. In advanced cases, kidney and placental impairment may occur.	Glucola test at 26 weeks. Go to GTT if > 140 mg%.	Diet, and in some cases, insulin.

Rh DISEASE

Definition	Symptoms	Diagnostic Tools	Treatment
Maternal Rh-antibodies cross the placenta and destroy the fetal blood cells, resulting in severe anemia and sometimes death of the fetus.		Rh testing	Prevention: The mother is given Rhogam injections at different intervals both during and following the pregnancy. This will keep her body from forming antibodies that will destroy the next baby's blood cells.

FETAL ALCOHOL SYNDROME

Definition	Symptoms	Diagnostic Tools	Treatment
A cluster of mental and physical birth defects.	The babies are usually smaller-than-normal, sicker-than-normal and are at greater risk to be stillborn; mental deficiencies may not show up for years.	Blood work	Treat the baby's symptoms. No cure.

(continued on following page)

4

OBSTETRICAL DISEASES AND DISORDERS *(continued from previous page)*

ECTOPIC PREGNANCY

Definition	Symptoms	Diagnostic Tools	Treatment
A pregnancy that occurs outside the uterus. Common sites include in the tube, cervix, ovary, abdominal or pelvic cavity. Can lead to rupture between weeks 12 and 15. This could lead to rapid hemorrhage and death.	Menstrual irregularities, spotting and cramping, pain and/or hemorrhage.	Ultrasound and needle aspiration; pregnancy test (Quantitative HCG should double.)	Methotrexate regimen

HYPEREMESIS GRAVIDARUM

Definition	Symptoms	Diagnostic Tools	Treatment
Nausea and vomiting that cause dehydration, weight loss, and acidosis.	Severe nausea and vomiting, weight loss, dehydration, jaundice, and an increase in pulse rate, retinitis, and hemorrhagic retinitis.	Usually tests are done to rule out other problems, like kidney and liver functioning. Ophthalmoscopic exams are done as well. Blood pH levels should be monitored.	IV infusion of water, glucose, and electrolytes. Sometimes antiemetics and sedatives are necessary. In severe cases, termination of pregnancy may be necessary.

ANEMIA IN PREGNANCY

Definition	Symptoms	Diagnostic Tools	Treatment
Hgb concentration < 10 gm/dl	Fatigue and pale skin	Complete blood count and folic acid level	Diet and iron supplements

OBSTETRICAL DIAGNOSTIC TESTS AND PROCEDURES

BLOOD TESTS

TEST NAME	DESCRIPTION	INDICATED CONDITION
Pregnancy Testing	Can be done on serum or urine. HCG can be detected in blood serum within a few days of conception. HCG can be detected in the urine usually within 5 days of the missed period.	Routinely done on women who suspect they are pregnant.
Complete Blood Count	Includes hemoglobin, hematocrit, WBC count, RBC count, differential, and platelet count.	Routine OB initial testing. Also done at different intervals on patients with suspected anemia.
Rh Factor and ABO Testing	Checks the exact blood type of the patient. Also checks to see if the patient has the Rh factor or not.	Routine OB initial testing
Rubella Titer	Checks the level of antibody against rubella (German measles), which is present in the patient's blood. Important because measles during pregnancy can cause congenital abnormalities (especially in the first trimester).	Routine OB initial testing
Hepatitis B	A test to see if the patient has ever been exposed to hepatitis B. Women who test positive have a greater incidence of preterm labor and spontaneous abortion.	Routine OB initial testing
VDRL or RPR	Screening tests for syphilis. The microbes which cause syphilis can cross the placenta and cause intrauterine death or congenital syphilis or other serious birth defects.	Routine OB initial testing
HIV	Test that checks to see if the HIV virus is present in the blood. This is the virus that causes AIDS. It also can pass through the placenta and cause the fetus to become infected.	Routine OB initial testing

(continued on following page)

4

OBSTETRICAL DIAGNOSTIC TESTS AND PROCEDURES *(continued from previous page)*

BLOOD TESTS

TEST NAME	DESCRIPTION	INDICATED CONDITION
Glucose Tolerance Test	This is a 1-4 hour test that is performed between 24 and 28 weeks of pregnancy. It is done to check for gestational diabetes.	Routine OB testing
Alpha-Fetoprotein Analysis	This test is done to detect neural tube damage, routinely done between 15 and 18 weeks' gestation. A decrease in AFP may indicate an increased risk of the baby's having Down's syndrome. An increase may indicate a greater chance of the baby having anencephaly or spina bifida.	Routine OB testing

Some physicians also may screen for toxoplasmosis, caused by *Toxoplasma gondii*, which can be very serious to the developing fetus.

ROUTINE CULTURES

TEST NAME	DESCRIPTION	INDICATED CONDITION
Gonorrhea Culture	Culture to look for gonorrhea. This could cause ophthalmia neonatorum in the newborn, which could result in blindness.	Routine initial OB testing, done later in pregnancy when gonorrhea is suspected.
Chlamydia	Culture to detect the presence of a bacteria known as chlamydia. A neonate who is born to a patient with chlamydia may contract pneumonia or neonatal conjunctivitis.	Routine initial OB testing, done later in pregnancy when chlamydia is suspected.
Pap Smear (Papanicolaou)	Done to see if there are any cell abnormalities such as uterine infections or cancer. (Not a culture.)	Routine initial OB testing

(continued on following page)

OBSTETRICAL DIAGNOSTIC TESTS AND PROCEDURES *(continued from previous page)*

OTHER OB DIAGNOSTIC TESTING

TEST NAME	DESCRIPTION	INDICATED CONDITION
Fundal Height Measurement	Provides an estimate of the duration of the pregnancy. Also gives the physician an idea of the development of the baby.	Done routinely at different intervals throughout the pregnancy.
Fetal Heart Tones	Used to figure the fetal heart rate. Normal fetal heart rate is between 120-160 beats per minute. If the heart rate falls below 120, it could mean fetal distress.	Done routinely after 8-10 weeks of gestation. Considered routine OB testing.
Amniocentesis	Can determine certain chromosomal abnormalities. Can also determine the sex of the baby.	Usually done on patients over the age of 35 or patients who have familial histories of chromosomal disorders. Routinely done on patients between the 14th and 16th week of pregnancy.
Fetal Heart Rate Monitoring (FHR)	Performed later in the pregnancy to detect any physical defects.	Done on patients with gestational diabetes, patients who complain of decreased fetal movement, patients who have decreased amniotic fluid, hypertensive obstetric patients, or if fetal growth is not progressing well or the patient is overdue.
Nonstress Test (NST) Part of the (FHR)	Detects changes in fetal heart rate when the baby moves. The baby's heart rate normally increases with movement.	Same as fetal heart rate monitoring
Contraction Stress Test (CST)	Checks to see what happens to the baby' heart rate when contractions are present. If CST is abnormal, further testing may be indicated.	Same as fetal heart rate monitoring
Obstetrical Ultrasound Testing	Allows the technician or doctor the ability to view the fetus and movement of the fetus.	Routinely done between weeks 16 and 22 to detect ectopic pregnancies, placental positioning, abnormal bleeding, presence of multiple fetuses, baby's position and size later in the pregnancy, and to evaluate fetal growth and confirm that the fetus is alive.

SECTION

5

PEDIATRICS

Introduction

Pediatrics is a rewarding profession, but it is not a field for everyone. To work in pediatrics, you must enjoy children and have a great deal of patience. You must be caring and empathetic, but not highly emotional, and you must possess a great deal of energy and have the ability to communicate with children from infancy through adolescence.

The pediatric section contains the following:

1. A Routine Procedure Chart: This is a sample chart that lists various procedures done at different age intervals. A blank form, the Pediatric Routine Procedures Form, can be found in Section 12. This form can be filled out and personalized to meet the specific needs of the office in which the assistant is working.

2. Summary of Rules of Childhood Immunizations: This chart lists the different age intervals when immunizations should be administered and important information about each immunization.

3. General Pediatric Assessment Form: This chart is designed to help the assistant who will be doing telephone triaging in a pediatric setting. It should not take the place of the assessment charts found in Section 3, but rather should alert the assistant with one quick glance as to which children should be seen and how quickly they should be seen. If this chart does not follow the general criteria of the office in which the assistant is currently working, a blank form, the General Pediatric Assessment Form, can be found in Section 12. The assistant can fill out the chart to meet the general guidelines of the office with which he or she is affiliated.

4. Common Pediatric Diseases and Disorders: This chart lists common pediatric diseases and disorders, defines each of the illnesses, lists the symptoms to look for, the usual treatments, and the possible diagnostic testing that may be needed for each.

PEDIATRIC ROUTINE PROCEDURES SAMPLE CHART

Age	HC	WT	HT	PP	LAB TESTS	ROUTINE PROCEDURES
NB	X	X	X	X	Newborn screening	Apgar scores, anticipatory guidance, safety issues, (circumcision for some males)
1 mo	X	X	X	X	Newborn screening	Anticipatory and nutrition guidance, accident prevention
2 mo	X	X	X	X		Anticipatory guidance
4 mo	X	X	X	X		Anticipatory guidance
6 mo	X	X	X	X	Optional (hematocrit and hemoglobin) for low birth weight babies	Anticipatory guidance
9 mo	X	X	X	X	Optional (hematocrit and hemoglobin) term babies	Anticipatory guidance, safety information, poison control kit from pharmacy
12 mo	X	X	X	X		Anticipatory guidance
15 mo	X	X	X	X		Anticipatory guidance
18 mo	X	X	X	X		Anticipatory guidance
4-6 yr		X	X	X	Optional urinalysis, hematocrit and hemoglobin	Vision and hearing screening, blood pressure, pulse and respiration
11-12 yr		X	X	X	Optional urinalysis, hematocrit and hemoglobin	Blood pressure, pulse and respiration
14-16 yr		X	X	X	Optional urinalysis, hematocrit and hemoglobin	Blood pressure, pulse and respiration

Abbreviations: HC-Head Circumference, WT-Weight, HT-Height, PP-Plot Percentiles

Any Modifications:

Physician's Approval:

IMMUNIZATION SCHEDULE

IMMUNIZATION ABBREVIATIONS

HBV	Hepatitis B virus vaccine	**HbCV**	Haemophilus influenzae b polysaccharide antigen conjugated to a special protein carrier
DTP	Diphtheria and tetanus toxoids with pertussis vaccine absorbed	**MMR**	Live measles, mumps, and rubella viruses vaccine
DTaP	Diphtheria and tetanus toxoids and acellular pertussis vaccine, absorbed	**OPV**	Live oral poliovirus vaccine
Td	Adult tetanus toxoid (full dose) and diphtheria toxoid (reduced dose)	**Varivox**	Varicella vaccine (chicken pox)
Hib	Haemophilus influenza type b conjugate vaccine		

Because immunization schedules change so rapidly and can differ from one office to another, a blank immunization chart that can be personalized according to the needs of your office is provided. It is recommended that the chart be filled out in pencil so that subsequent changes can be made as necessary.

SCHEDULE

Newborn						
2 months						
4 months						
6 months						
12 months						
15 months						
18 months						
2-6 years						
12 years						
14-16 years						
Additional age ranges						

Any Modifications: _____

Physician's Approval: _____

GENERAL PEDIATRIC ASSESSMENT SAMPLE CHART

Call EMS	Should Be Seen in Office ASAP	(Same Day—24 Hours)	(Within the Week)
Any life-threatening injuries	Abdominal pain (acute), especially if right-sided, or if other Sx are present.	Abdominal pain (chronic), s̄ any other Sx	Behavioral or emotional problems
Any life-threatening illnesses	Asthma (acute attack), but not severe.	Cold Sx c̄ fever > 100° F	Routine check-ups
Anaphylactic reactions (e.g., bee stings)	Burns on genitals, buttocks, hands, feet, or face, loose or charred skin, blisters present over 2" in diameter.	Diarrhea (chronic) s̄ any other Sx	Routine general concerns
Asthma (severe attacks)	Cough that is productive or in association c̄ fever or breathing problems.	Fever < 101° F under age of 6 mo. (No other Sx)	Usual follow-up exams
Breathing difficulties	Croup, if in conjunction with other Sx.	Fever < 103° F over the age of 6 mo.	
Burns that are severe	Diarrhea (acute) > than 4-6 stools in 12-hour period, or connected c̄ acute pain or high fever.	Fever connected to chronic illness	
Hemorrhaging	Dehydration cases	Headache (chronic) s̄ other Sx	
Poisonous substance ingestion	Ear pain	Prescription renewals	
Seizure (1st time)	Eye infections or eye injuries	Rash (persistent diaper rash)	
Shock	Fever > 101° F if under the age of 6 mo.	Rash (asymptomatic)	
Unconscious patient	Fever > 103° F if over the age of 6 mo.	Seizure (follow-up if no current Sx are present)	
	Fever > 100° F if in conjunction c̄ acute illness.	Stomach upset, s̄ any other Sx	
	Headache (migraine variant)	Stools (blood c̄ no other Sx)	
	Headache, with high fever, stiff neck, visual disturbances, vomiting, or strange behavior.	Strains (mild pain)	
	Insect bites or stings that look suspicious or infected (any insect or animal bite).	Urinary Sx (chronic back pain or fever)	

(continued on following page)

GENERAL PEDIATRIC ASSESSMENT SAMPLE CHART *(continued from previous page)*

Call EMS	Should Be Seen in Office ASAP	(Same Day—24 Hours)	(Within the Week)
Unconscious patient	Lacerations that are gaping, other wounds that might be infected, dog bites that break the skin, or any red streaks that run upward from a wound.	Vomiting (mild in nature) s̄ severe pain or high fever	
	Poison follow-ups (if directed by Poison Control Center).		
	Rashes that are in conjunction c̄ fever, earache, sore throat, or that might be related to a medication.		
	Sore throat c̄ fever > 100° F, pus patches, swollen glands, stiff neck, or acting very ill.		
	Sprains or strains (possible), very painful		
	Unconscious (patient was unconscious and is now conscious)		
	Urinary symptoms, if in conjunction with fever, back pain, or vomiting, vaginal or penile discharge.		
	Vomiting (severe) or blood present, or persisting > 24 hours.		

Any Modifications:

Physician's Approval: _____

COMMON PEDIATRIC DISEASES AND DISORDERS

DISEASE: OTITIS MEDIA

DEFINITION	SYMPTOMS	USUAL TREATMENT
A bacterial or viral infection of the middle ear. Usually secondary to a URI. Most common in ages 3 months to 3 years.	Severe earache, fever, nausea/vomiting, and diarrhea. May have a discharge when tympanic membrane is ruptured.	Antibiotic therapy, i.e., amoxicillin

DISEASE: STREPTOCOCCAL PHARYNGITIS

DEFINITION	SYMPTOMS	USUAL TREATMENT
Invasion of streptococcus in the throat region.	Will vary. Sore throat, may have erythema, and/or pustules, high fever, possible rash.	Antibiotic therapy i.e., penicillin (G or V)

POSSIBLE LABS: THROAT CULTURE/RAPID STREP TEST

DISEASE: ASTHMA

DEFINITION	SYMPTOMS	USUAL TREATMENT
A lung disease characterized by (1) airway(s) obstruction that is reversible; (2) airway(s) inflammation, and (3) increase in airway(s) responsiveness to a variety of stimuli.	Will vary. Some airway obstruction of varying degree, hyperventilation, mild coughing and wheezing, inability to speak, fatigue, cyanosis, severe distress, confusion, and lethargy.	Will vary. Bronchodilators; drug therapy may include any of the following: beta-adrenergic agents, theophylline, corticosteroids, cromolyn sodium, and anti-cholinergic agents.

POSSIBLE DIAGNOSTIC TESTING (May include any of the following): Blood ABG and sputum analysis, chest Xray, pulmonary function testing, and lung sounds.

DISEASE: GASTROENTERITIS

DEFINITION	SYMPTOMS	USUAL TREATMENT
A syndrome of vomiting and diarrhea caused by pathogenic microorganisms that may lead to dehydration and an electrolyte imbalance.	Will vary, but may include any of the following: diarrhea, vomiting, and dehydration, Sx such as lethargy, anorexia, fever, oliguria, and marked weight loss.	Rehydration therapy; antibiotic therapy in bacterial infections

DIAGNOSTIC TESTING (May include any of the following): Hematocrit, serum electrolytes, urinalysis, stool cultures, and CBC.

(continued on following page)

COMMON PEDIATRIC DISEASES AND DISORDERS *(continued from previous page)*

DISEASE: PNEUMONIA

DEFINITION	SYMPTOMS	USUAL TREATMENT
Acute infection of the lung parenchyma including the alveolar spaces and interstitial tissue. Usually secondary to an upper respiratory infection.	Will vary, but may include fever, pain upon breathing, dyspnea, chills, cough, sputum production, an increase in pulse and respiration, nausea, vomiting, malaise, and myalgias.	Antibiotic therapy, i.e., penicillin G, possible inhalation therapy

DIAGNOSTIC TESTING (May include any of the following): Chest Xray and sputum analysis.

DISEASE: UPPER RESPIRATORY INFECTION

DEFINITION	SYMPTOMS	USUAL TREATMENT
Viral infection of the respiratory tract with inflammation in any or all of the airways.	Nasal or throat discomfort followed by sneezing, rhinorrhea, and malaise.	Rest, analgesics, nasal decongestants, and antihistamines

DIAGNOSTIC TESTING (May include any or all the following): Physical assessment and smear of any exudates.

DISEASE: URINARY TRACT INFECTION

DEFINITION	SYMPTOMS	USUAL TREATMENT
Invasion of bacteria in the urinary tract. May be asymptomatic or with the manifestation of cystitis or pyelonephritis.	Will vary, but may include dysuria, urinary frequency, hematuria, urinary retention, supra-pubic pain, urinary incontinence, or foul-smelling urine.	Antibiotics and lots of water

DIAGNOSTIC TESTING (May include any or all of the following): Urinalysis, culture, and sensitivity.

(continued on following page)

COMMON PEDIATRIC DISEASES AND DISORDERS *(continued from previous page)*

DISEASE: IMPETIGO

DEFINITION	SYMPTOMS	USUAL TREATMENT
A superficial vesiculopustular skin infection that is usually caused from a break in the skin's surface or irritation of the nostril from a runny nose.	Lesions that may be located on the arms, legs, and face. Lesions may be anywhere from the size of a pea to very large. Exudate may be present and may crust over. Some itching may be present.	Systemic antibiotics and topical antibiotics

DISEASE: ECZEMA

DEFINITION	SYMPTOMS	USUAL TREATMENT
Superficial skin inflammation that occurs in children who have a genetic tendency toward allergies	Inflamed skin characterized by vesicles, redness, edema, oozing, crusting, scaling. Itching may be a problem as well.	Removal of offending agent; oral and/or topical corticosteriods may also be used.

DIAGNOSTIC TESTING: Patch testing

DIAGNOSIS: PITYRIASIS ROSEA

DEFINITION	SYMPTOMS	USUAL TREATMENT
A self-limited, mild, inflammatory skin disease characterized by scaly lesions, possibly due to an unidentified infectious agent.	A "Herald Patch" or "Mother Patch" commonly found on the trunk. It is slightly erythematous and rose- or fawn-colored. It has a slightly raised border and resembles ringworm. Similar lesions may occur that can be anywhere from 0.5 to 2.0 centimeters in diameter. Patient may have some itching.	Usually none. Sunlight may help. Prednisone may be used in cases where itching is a major factor.

DIAGNOSTIC TESTING: Serological test for syphilis may be performed because the lesions can resemble those that occur with secondary syphilis.

(continued on following page)

COMMON PEDIATRIC DISEASES AND DISORDERS *(continued from previous page)*

DISEASE: DIAPER DERMATITIS

DEFINITION

A rash that can appear anywhere in the groin region or in the gluteal folds of the buttocks. It usually starts from a moist diaper that rubs against the skin. The rash may become infected with bacteria or yeast.

SYMPTOMS

Skin will have patches of erythematous tissue which sometimes contain exudative patches varying in size and shape. Red base pustules may occur.

USUAL TREATMENT

Air-drying the skin can help the rash, as can changing the diaper often and applying a protective barrier like Vaseline or Desitin.

DISEASE: SCABIES

DEFINITION

Caused by the itch mite *Sarcoptes scabiei*. The impregnated female mite tunnels her way into the epidermis and deposits her eggs along the burrow. Larvae hatch within a few days and congregate along the hair follicle.

SYMPTOMS

Severe itching, which is intensified when the patient is in a supine position. Initial lesions are burrows that have fine, wavy, dark lines anywhere from a few millimeters to 1 centimeter long, with a minute papule at the open end. Lesions occur on the finger webs, wrists, elbows, axillary folds, trunk, and extremities.

USUAL TREATMENT

5% permethrin cream; the whole family should be treated.

DISEASE: PINWORMS *(ENTEROBIUS VERMICULARIS)*

DEFINITION

Small, white, threadlike worms that may enter the body through the oral route from food or from placing contaminated objects in the mouth. Eggs hatch in the intestines, where they quickly become adult worms and multiply rapidly. Female worms lay eggs near the anus at night, causing itching. The child scratches and picks up eggs on the fingers. The oral fecal route is established; others are soon infected. Direct transfer of eggs is from the anus to the mouth; indirectly with eggs in clothing and bedding.

SYMPTOMS

Severe anal itching, increased hunger, stomach ache, restless sleep; observing worms around the anus during the night with a flashlight or before BM (also, irritability).

USUAL TREATMENT

Oral medication for the entire family; topical medication for anal irritation; scrupulous hygiene; shorten fingernails; launder items in hottest water possible.

VISUAL IDENTIFICATION GUIDE

Use this section to quickly verify the identity of a capsule, tablet, or other solid oral medication. More than 200 leading products are shown in actual size and color, organized alphabetically by generic name. Each product is labeled with its brand name, if applicable, as well as its strength and the name of its supplier.

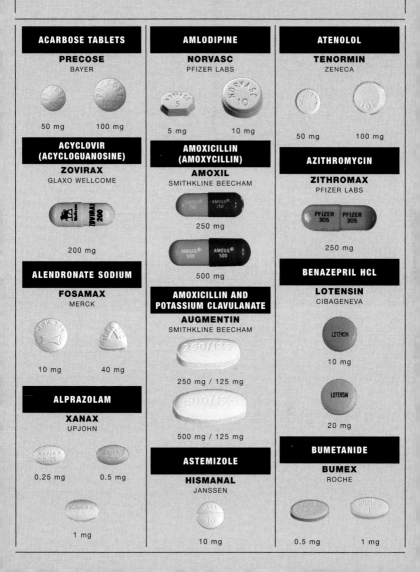

ACARBOSE TABLETS
PRECOSE
BAYER

50 mg   100 mg

ACYCLOVIR (ACYCLOGUANOSINE)
ZOVIRAX
GLAXO WELLCOME

200 mg

ALENDRONATE SODIUM
FOSAMAX
MERCK

10 mg   40 mg

ALPRAZOLAM
XANAX
UPJOHN

0.25 mg   0.5 mg

1 mg

AMLODIPINE
NORVASC
PFIZER LABS

5 mg   10 mg

AMOXICILLIN (AMOXYCILLIN)
AMOXIL
SMITHKLINE BEECHAM

250 mg

500 mg

AMOXICILLIN AND POTASSIUM CLAVULANATE
AUGMENTIN
SMITHKLINE BEECHAM

250 mg / 125 mg

500 mg / 125 mg

ASTEMIZOLE
HISMANAL
JANSSEN

10 mg

ATENOLOL
TENORMIN
ZENECA

50 mg   100 mg

AZITHROMYCIN
ZITHROMAX
PFIZER LABS

250 mg

BENAZEPRIL HCL
LOTENSIN
CIBAGENEVA

10 mg

20 mg

BUMETANIDE
BUMEX
ROCHE

0.5 mg   1 mg

BUSPIRONE HCL

BUSPAR
BRISTOL-MYERS SQUIBB

5 mg

10 mg

CAPTOPRIL

CAPOTEN
BRISTOL-MYERS SQUIBB

12.5 mg

25 mg

50 mg

CARBAMAZEPINE

TEGRETOL
CIBAGENEVA

200 mg

CEFACLOR

CECLOR
ELI LILLY

250 mg

500 mg

CEFADROXIL MONOHYDRATE

DURICEF
BRISTOL-MYERS SQUIBB

500 mg

CEFIXIME

SUPRAX
LEDERLE

400 mg

CEFPROZIL

CEFZIL
BRISTOL-MYERS SQUIBB

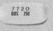

250 mg

CEFUROXIME AXETIL

CEFTIN
GLAXO

250 mg

500 mg

CIMETIDINE

TAGAMET
SMITHKLINE BEECHAM

300 mg

400 mg

CIPROFLOXACIN HCL

CIPRO
BAYER

250 mg

500 mg

CLARITHROMYCIN

BIAXIN
ABBOTT

250 mg

500 mg

CLONAZEPAM

KLONOPIN
ROCHE

0.5 mg   1 mg

CYCLOBENZAPRINE HCL

FLEXERIL
MERCK

10 mg

DARVOCET-N 100

ACETAMINOPHEN AND PROPOXYPHENE NAPSYLATE
ELI LILLY

650 mg / 100 mg

DIAZEPAM

VALIUM
ROCHE

2 mg

5 mg

10 mg

DICLOFENAC SODIUM

VOLTAREN
CIBAGENEVA

50 mg   75 mg

DICYCLOMINE HCL

BENTYL
HOECHST MARION ROUSSEL

10 mg

20 mg

DIGOXIN

LANOXIN
BURROUGHS WELLCOME

0.125 mg   0.25 mg

DILTIAZEM HCL

CARDIZEM CD
HOECHST MARION ROUSSEL

120 mg

180 mg

240 mg

DIVALPROEX SODIUM

DEPAKOTE
ABBOTT

250 mg

500 mg

DOXAZOSIN MESYLATE

CARDURA
ROERIG

1 mg   2 mg

ENALAPRIL MALEATE

VASOTEC
MERCK

5 mg   10 mg

20 mg

ERYTHROMYCIN BASE

ERY-TAB
ABBOTT

250 mg

333 mg

ERYTHROMYCIN
ABBOTT

250 mg

PCE
ABBOTT

333 mg

500 mg

ERYTHROMYCIN STEARATE

ERYTHROCIN STEARATE FILMTAB
ABBOTT

250 mg

500 mg

ESTROGENS CONJUGATED

PREMARIN
WYETH-AYERST

0.3 mg   0.625 mg

1.25 mg

ESTROPIPATE (PIPERAZINE ESTRONE SULFATE)

OGEN
UPJOHN

0.625 mg

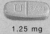

1.25 mg

ETODOLAC

LODINE
WYETH-AYERST

300 mg

400 mg

FAMOTIDINE

PEPCID
MERCK

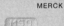

20 mg   40 mg

FINASTERIDE

PROSCAR
MERCK

5 mg

FIORINAL

BUTALBITAL AND ASPIRIN AND CAFFEINE
SANDOZ

50 mg / 325 mg / 40 mg

50 mg / 325 mg / 40 mg

FLUOXETINE HCL

PROZAC
DISTA

10 mg

20 mg

FLURBIPROFEN

ANSAID
UPJOHN

50 mg

100 mg

FOSINOPRIL SODIUM

MONOPRIL
BRISTOL-MYERS SQUIBB

10 mg   20 mg

FUROSEMIDE

LASIX
HOECHST MARION ROUSSEL

20 mg   40 mg

GEMFIBROZIL

LOPID
PARKE-DAVIS

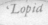

600 mg

GLIPIZIDE

GLUCOTROL
PRATT

5 mg   10 mg

GLYBURIDE

DIABETA
HOECHST MARION ROUSSEL

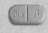

2.5 mg   5 mg

GLYNASE PRESTAB
UPJOHN

3 mg

MICRONASE
UPJOHN

2.5 mg   5 mg

GUANFACINE HCL

TENEX
A. H. ROBINS

1 mg

HYDROCODONE BITARTRATE AND ACETAMINOPHEN

VICODIN
KNOLL

5 mg / 500 mg

IBUPROFEN	KETOCONAZOLE	LORACARBEF

IBUPROFEN
MOTRIN
UPJOHN

400 mg

600 mg

800 mg

INDAPAMIDE
LOZOL
RHONE-POULENC RORER

1.25 mg   2.5 mg

ISOSORBIDE DINITRATE TABLETS
ISORDIL TITRADOSE
WYETH-AYERST

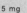
5 mg   10 mg

ISRADIPINE
DYNACIRC
SANDOZ

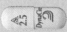
2.5 mg

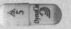
5 mg

KETOCONAZOLE
NIZORAL
JANSSEN

200 mg

KETOROLAC TROMETHAMINE
TORADOL
SYNTEX

10 mg

LEVOTHYROXINE SODIUM
SYNTHROID
KNOLL

0.05 mg   0.1 mg

0.15 mg

LISINOPRIL
PRINIVIL
MERCK

10 mg   20 mg

LISINOPRIL
ZESTRIL
ZENECA

5 mg

10 mg

20 mg

LORACARBEF
LORABID
ELI LILLY

200 mg

LORATADINE
CLARITIN
SCHERING

10 mg

LORAZEPAM
ATIVAN
WYETH-AYERST

0.5 mg   1 mg

LOSARTAN POTASSIUM
COZAAR
MERCK

25 mg   50 mg

LOVASTATIN (MEVINOLIN)
MEVACOR
MERCK

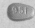
10 mg   20 mg

MEDROXYPROGESTERONE ACETATE
PROVERA
UPJOHN

2.5 mg   10 mg

METFORMIN HCL

GLUCOPHAGE
BRISTOL-MYERS SQUIBB

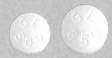

500 mg   850 mg

METHYLPHENIDATE HCL

RITALIN
CIBAGENEVA

5 mg   10 mg

METHYLPREDNISOLONE

MEDROL
UPJOHN

4 mg

METOPROLOL TARTRATE

LOPRESSOR
CIBAGENEVA

50 mg   100 mg

MISOPROSTOL

CYTOTEC
G. D. SEARLE

100 mcg   200 mcg

NABUMETONE

RELAFEN
SMITHKLINE BEECHAM

500 mg

NADOLOL

CORGARD
BRISTOL-MYERS SQUIBB

40 mg   80 mg

NAPROXEN

NAPROSYN
ROCHE

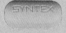

375 mg

500 mg

NAPROXEN SODIUM

ANAPROX
ROCHE

275 mg

ANAPROX DS
ROCHE

550 mg

NEFAZODONE HCL

SERZONE
BRISTOL-MYERS SQUIBB

100 mg

200 mg

NIFEDIPINE

PROCARDIA XL
PRATT

30 mg   60 mg

90 mg

NIZATIDINE

AXID
ELI LILLY

150 mg

NORTRIPTYLINE HCL

PAMELOR
SANDOZ

25 mg

50 mg

OFLOXACIN

FLOXIN
MCNEIL

300 mg

OMEPRAZOLE

PRILOSEC
ASTRA MERCK

20 mg

OXAPROZIN

DAYPRO
G. D. SEARLE

600 mg

OXYCODONE AND ACETAMINOPHEN

PERCOCET
DUPONT

5 mg / 325 mg

PAROXETINE HCL

PAXIL
SMITHKLINE BEECHAM

20 mg

PENICILLIN V POTASSIUM (PHENOXYMETHYL PENICILLIN POTASSIUM)

PEN-VEE K
WYETH-AYERST

250 mg   500 mg

PENTOXIFYLLINE

TRENTAL
HOECHST MARION ROUSSEL

400 mg

PHENYTOIN SODIUM, EXTENDED

DILANTIN KAPSEALS
PARKE-DAVIS

100 mg

POTASSIUM CHLORIDE

K-DUR
KEY

10 mEq

20 mEq

KLOR-CON 10
UPSHER-SMITH

10 mEq

MICRO-K 10 EXTENCAPS
A. H. ROBINS

10 mEq

PRAVASTATIN SODIUM

PRAVACHOL
BRISTOL-MYERS SQUIBB

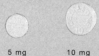

20 mg

PREDNISONE

DELTASONE
UPJOHN

5 mg   10 mg

20 mg

PROPRANOLOL HCL

INDERAL
WYETH-AYERST

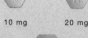

10 mg   20 mg

40 mg

INDERAL LA
WYETH-AYERST

80 mg

QUINAPRIL HCL

ACCUPRIL
PARKE-DAVIS

10 mg   20 mg

RAMIPRIL

ALTACE
HOECHST MARION ROUSSEL

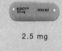

2.5 mg

5 mg

RANITIDINE HCL

ZANTAC
GLAXO

150 mg

300 mg

SERTRALINE HCL

ZOLOFT
ROERIG

50 mg

100 mg

SIMVASTATIN

ZOCOR
MERCK

10 mg   20 mg

SUCRALFATE

CARAFATE
HOECHST MARION ROUSSEL

1 gm

TAMOXIFEN

NOLVADEX
ZENECA

10 mg

TEMAZEPAM

RESTORIL
SANDOZ

15 mg

30 mg

TERAZOSIN

HYTRIN
ABBOTT

2 mg   5 mg

TERFENADINE

SELDANE
HOECHST MARION ROUSSEL

60 mg

TERFENADINE AND PSEUDOEPHEDRINE HCL

SELDANE-D
HOECHST MARION ROUSSEL

60 mg / 120 mg

THEOPHYLLINE

THEO-DUR
KEY

200 mg   300 mg

TRIAMTERENE AND HYDROCHLOROTHIAZIDE TABLETS

MAXZIDE
LEDERLE

37.5 mg/   75 mg/
25 mg   50 mg

TRIAMTERENE AND HYDROCHLOROTHIAZIDE CAPSULES

DYAZIDE
SMITHKLINE BEECHAM

 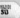

37.5 mg / 25 mg

TRIAZOLAM

HALCION
UPJOHN

0.125 mg   0.25 mg

TRIMETHOPRIM AND SULFAMETHOXAZOLE

BACTRIM DS
ROCHE

160 mg / 800 mg

TYLENOL WITH CODEINE TABLETS

ACETAMINOPHEN AND CODEINE PHOSPHATE
MCNEIL

300 mg / 30 mg

VERAPAMIL

CALAN SR
G. D. SEARLE

240 mg

WARFARIN SODIUM

COUMADIN
DUPONT PHARMA

2 mg

2.5 mg

5 mg

SECTION

6

MEDICATIONS

Prescription Abbreviations

$\overline{aa}$	of each	on	every night
ac	before meals	os	mouth
ad lib	as desired	oz	ounce
alt dieb	every other day	pc	after meals
alt hor	every other hour	po	by mouth, orally
alt noc	every other night	PRN	as needed
aq	aqueous (water)	qd	every day
bid	twice a day	qh	every hour
cap	capsule	q2h	every second hour
comp	compound	q3h	every third hour
dil	dilute	qid	four times a day
ELIX	elixir	ql	as much as is desired
g	gram	qn	every night
gr	grain	R	take
gt	drop	rep	let it be repeated
gtt	drops	$\overline{s}$	without
h	hour	seq	that which follows
hs	at bedtime	Sig	label; write; let it be written
M	mix; minimum	SOS	if necessary
noc	night	sp	spirit
non rep	do not repeat	ss	one-half
o	pint	STAT	immediately
OD	every other day	syr	syrup
oh	at every hour	tid	three times a day
ol	oil	tr/tinc	tincture
om	on every morning	ung	ointment

PARTS OF THE PRESCRIPTION

PHYSICIAN'S INFORMATION	PATIENT INFORMATION	MEDICATION INSTRUCTIONS
Physician's full name	Patient's full name	Superscription: The symbol "RX" comes from the Latin word *recipe* and means to "take."
Physician's address	Patient's full address	Inscription: The main portion of the order includes the name of the drug, dosage form, i.e., capsule, tablets, etc., and the dosage amount.
Physician's telephone number	Patient's age (when applicable)	Subscription: Includes any special instructions to the pharmacist and the amount to be dispensed ("Disp"). Some pharmacists require that the amount to be dispensed be both in numeric and written form, so no one can change the information.
Physician's DEA # (when applicable)		Signature: Latin abbreviation for *signetur*, means "write on label." Appears as "Sig" on the prescription form. It states when the patient is to take the medication, how often, any food precautions, and any storage information.
Physician's signature		Refills: The number of refills allowed.

Other miscellaneous information should include the date that it is issued and whether or not a generic is acceptable. Remember that in cases where the assistant is permitted to write the prescription, it must still always be signed by the physician.

(continued on following page)

PARTS OF THE PRESCRIPTION (continued from previous page)

PRESCRIPTION EXAMPLE

Walter E. Allen, M. D.
345 E. Molar Rd.
Columbus, OH 43207
555-0500

Patient's Name: _____ Age: _____

Address: _____ Date: _____

(Superscription) RX

(Inscription) *Amoxicillin 250 mg caps*

(Subscription) *Disp: # 30 (Thirty)*

(Signature) *Sig: 1 cap po tid x 10 days*

Generic Equivalent OK _____

Any Refills: None, 1, 2, 3, 4, 5

Physician's Signature: _____

DEA #: _____

DRUG CLASSIFICATIONS

CLASSIFICATION	ACTION	EXAMPLES
Analgesic	Relieves pain	Narcotic: morphine, codeine Non-narcotic: aspirin, acetaminophen
Anesthetic	Produces a lack of feeling (can be local or general)	Lidocaine, Procaine
Angiotensin-Converting Enzyme Inhibitor (Ace-Inhibitor)	Suppresses the renin-angiotensin aldosterone system. Leads to sodium and fluid loss and therefore a drop in blood pressure.	Captopril, Lisinopril
Antacid	Neutralizes stomach acid	Mylanta, Maalox, Gaviscon
Antiacne	Prevents or works against acne	Retin A
Antianemic	Prevents/treats anemia	Niferex-PN, Theragran
Antianginal	Dilates blood vessels of the heart and reduces cardiac oxygen demand	Nitrostat, Procardia
Antianxiety	Relieves anxiety and muscle tension	Valium, Librium
Antiarrhythmic	Controls cardiac arrhythmias	Inderal, Quinidine
Antiasthmatic	A drug used to treat asthma patients	Intal, Slo-Bid
Antibiotic	Destructive to or inhibits the growth of microorgansims	Augmentin, Unipen, Keflin
Anticholinergic	Reduces gastric motility by antagonizing the action of acetylcholine in the parasympathetic nervous system (also known as antispasmodic)	Atropine, Scopolamine
Anticoagulant	Prevents or delays blood clotting	Coumadin, Heparin Sodium
Anticonvulsant	Prevents or relieves convulsions	Dilantin, Zarontin
Antidepressant	Prevents or relieves symptoms of depression	Prozac, Triavil
Antidiarrheal	Prevents or relieves diarrhea	Lomotil, Kaopectate
Antidote	Counteracts poisons and their effects	Antilirium

(continued on following page)

DRUG CLASSIFICATIONS *(continued from previous page)*

CLASSIFICATION	ACTION	EXAMPLES
Antiemetic	Prevents or relieves nausea and vomiting	Phenergan, Tigan
Antifungal	Kills or prevents the growth of fungi and yeast	Monistat, Nizoral
Antihistamine	Counteracts histamine production	Benadryl, Tavist
Antihyperlipidemic	Agents that help to decrease elevated and total LDH cholesterol	Lovastatin, Mevacor
Antihypertensive	Prevents or controls hypertension	Esidrix, Lopressor
Anti-infective	Antibiotic therapy to prevent secondary infections	Loracarbef, Vancomycin
Anti-inflammatory	An agent that counteracts inflammation	Aspirin, Feldene, Motrin
Antiulcer	Inhibits histamine, thereby decreasing gastric secretion or forming a barrier at the ulcer site	Tagamet, Zantac
Benzodiazepine	Minor tranquilizers, most widely prescribed for the treatment of anxiety	Xanax, Ativan
Beta-Adrenergic Agent (Beta-Blocker)	Blocks the response to sympathetic nerve impulses; useful in treating conditions like hypertension, cardiac arrhythmias, MIs, and migraines	Atenolol, Timolol Maleate
Bronchodilator	Dilates the bronchi	Isuprel, Ventolin
Ca-Channel Blocking Agents	Inhibits the influx of calcium ions into myocardial muscle and myocardial pacemaker cells and helps produce antianginal and antihypertensive effects	Verapamil
Cardiac Glycosides	Plant alkaloids; most effective for treating congestive heart failure	Digitoxin, Digoxin
Cardiotonic	Increases the strength of the heart muscle	Lanoxin, Digitoxin
Contraceptive	Prevents conception	Triphasil, Ovrette

(continued on following page)

DRUG CLASSIFICATIONS *(continued from previous page)*

CLASSIFICATION	ACTION	EXAMPLES
Corticosteroids	Hormones that are naturally manufactured by the adrenal gland; can be made synthetically and used for anti-inflammatory or immunosuppressant therapy	Prednisone, Betamethasone
Cough Expectorant	An agent that helps to liquify mucus and promote its removal	Robitussin, Triaminic Expectorant
Cough Suppressant (Antitussive)	Depresses the cough reflex which is located in the medulla of the brain	Narcotic: Simetane-DC Syrup Non-narcotic: Tuss-Ornade
Decongestant	Reduces nasal congestion/swelling	Comtrex, Naldecon
Diuretic	Increases the excretion of urine	Dyazide, Lasix
Emetic	Facilitates vomiting	Syrup of Ipecac
Hemostatic	Controls or stops bleeding	Thrombostat, Amicar
Histamine H$_2$ Receptor Antagonist	Blocks all phases of gastric acid secretion (antacid)	Cimetidine, Rantidine
Hypnotic	Produces sleep or hypnosis	Dalmane, Placidyl
Hypoglycemic (Antidiabetic)	Lowers blood glucose level	Micronase, Glucotrol
Laxative	Loosens and promotes normal bowel eliminations	Fibercon, Dialose Plus
Muscle Relaxant	Aids in relaxation of skeletal muscles	Norflex, Robaxin, Soma
NSAID	Nonsteroidal anti-inflammatory drug (anti-inflammatory)	Naproxen, Ketoprofen
Sedative	Produces a calming effect	Phenobarbital, Benadryl
Tranquilizer	Reduces mental tension and anxiety	Ativan, Xanax
Vasodilator	Produces relaxation of blood vessels; lowers blood pressure	Nitro Bid, Isordil
Vasopressor	Produces contraction of blood vessels; elevates blood pressure	Aramine, Intropin

MOST COMMONLY PRESCRIBED BRAND-NAME MEDICATIONS

Medications indicated with an asterisk (*) appear in the drug insert.

TRADE NAME	GENERIC	CLASSIFICATION	SCHEDULE
*Accupril	Quinapril hydrochloride	Antihypertensive	
Adalat CC	Nifedipine	Antianginal, antihypertensive	
*Altace	Ramipril	Antihypertensive	
Ambien	Zolpidem tartrate	Sedative-hypnotic	(C-IV)
*Amoxil	Amoxicillin	Antibiotic (Penicillin)	
*Ansaid	Flurbiprofen	NSAID	
*Ativan	Lorazepam	Antianxiety	(C-IV)
Atrovent	Ipratropium bromide	Bronchodilator (anticholinergic)	
*Augmentin	Amoxicillin and potassium clavulanate	Antibiotic (Penicillin)	
*Axid	Nizatidine	Histamine H_2 receptor antagonist	
Azmacort	Triamcinolone acetonide	Corticosteroid anti-inflammatory	
Bactroban	Mupirocin	Topical anti-infective	
Beconase AQ	Beclomethasone dipropionate	Glucocorticoid	
*Bentyl	Dicyclomine HCL	Antispasmodic, cholinergicblocking agent	
*Biaxin	Clarithromycin	Antibiotic	
*Bumex	Bumetanide	Loop diuretic	
*Buspar	Buspirone hydrochloride	Antianxiety	
*Calan SR	Verapamil hydrochloride	Antihypertensive (Ca-blocker)	
*Capoten	Captopril	Antihypertensive	
*Carafate	Sucralfate	Antiulcer	
*Cardizem CD	Diltiazem hydrochloride	Antianginal, antihypertensive	
*Cardura	Doxazosin mesylate	Antihypertensive	

(continued on following page)

MOST COMMONLY PRESCRIBED BRAND-NAME MEDICATIONS *(continued from previous page)*

TRADE NAME	GENERIC	CLASSIFICATION	SCHEDULE
*Ceclor	Cefaclor	Cephalosporin (second-generation)	
*Ceftin	Cefuroxime axetil	Cephalosporin (second-generation)	
*Cefzil	Cefprozil	Cephalosporin (second-generation)	
*Cipro	Ciprofloxacin	Anti-infective	
*Claritin	Loratadine pseudophedrine sulfate	Antihistamine	
Compazine	Prochlorperazine	Antipsychotic, antiemetic	
*Corgard	Nadolol	Antihypertensive/antianginal	
Cotrim	Trimethoprim, sulfamethoxazole	Antibiotic	
*Coumadin	Warfarin sodium	Anticoagulant	
*Cozaar	Losartan potassium	Antihypertensive	
Cycrin	Medroxyprogesterone acetate	Progestational hormone	
*Cytotec	Misoprostol	Antiulcer	
*Darvocet-N 100	Propoxyphene napsylate, acetaminophen	Narcotic and non-narcotic analgesic	(C-IV)
*DayPro	Oxaprozin	NSAID	
Demulen 1/35-28	Ethynodiol diacetate, ethinyl estradiol	Oral contraceptive	
*Depakote	Divalproex sodium	Anticonvulsant	
Desogen	Desogestrel and ethinyl estradiol	Oral contraceptive	
*DiaBeta	Glyburide	Antidiabetic	
Dilacor XR	Diltiazem hydrochloride	Antianginal, antihypertensive	
Dilantin	Phenytoin	Anticonvulsant, antiarrhythmic	
*Duricef	Cefadroxil monohydrate	Cephalosporin (first-generation)	
Dyazide	Hydrochlorothiazide, triamterene	Diuretic, antihypertensive	
*DynaCirc	Isradipine	Antihypertensive (Ca-channel blocker)	

(continued on following page)

MOST COMMONLY PRESCRIBED BRAND-NAME MEDICATIONS *(continued from previous page)*

TRADE NAME	GENERIC	CLASSIFICATION	SCHEDULE
E.E.S.	Erythromycin ethylsuccinate	Anti-infective	
EFFEXOR	Venlafaxine hydrochloride	Antidepressant	
Elocon	Mometasone furoate	Steroidal anti-inflammatory	
Entex LA	Phenylpropanolamine hydrochloride, guaifenesin	Expectorant, decongestant	
*Ery-Tab	Erythromycin base	Antibiotic (Erythromycin)	
*Erythromycin	Erythromycin base	Antibiotic (Erythromycin)	
*Erythrocin Stearate	Erythromycin stearate	Antibiotic (Erythromycin)	
Estrace	Estradiol	Estrogen hormone	
Estraderm	Estradiol transdermal system	Estrogen hormone	
Feldene	Piroxicam	NSAID	
Flonase	Fluticasone dipropionate	Steroidal anti-inflammatory	
*Floxin	Ofloxacin	Antibacterial	
Fosamax	Alendronate sodium	Antipostmenopausal osteoporosis	
Glucophage	Metformin	Antidiabetic	
*Glucotrol	Glipizide	Antidiabetic	
*Glynase PresTab	Glyburide	Antidiabetic	
*Halcion	Triazolam	Sedative/Hypnotic	(C-IV)
*Hismanal	Astemizole	Antihistamine	
Humulin N	Human insulin	Insulin	
Humulin R	Human insulin	Rapid-acting insulin	
Humulin 70/30	Human insulin	Insulin	
*Hytrin	Terazosin	Antihypertensive	
Imitrex	Sumatriptan succinate	Antimigraine	

(continued on following page)

MOST COMMONLY PRESCRIBED BRAND-NAME MEDICATIONS (continued from previous page)

TRADE NAME	GENERIC	CLASSIFICATION	SCHEDULE
*Inderal	Propranolol hydrochloride	Antihypertensive, antianginal	
Inderal-LA	Propranolol (extended release)	Antihypertensive	
Intal	Cromolyn sodium	Antiasthmatic, antiallergic	
*K-Dur	Potassium chloride	Electrolyte	
Keflex	Cephalexin	Antibiotic	
*Klonopin	Clonazepam	Anticonvulsant	(C-IV)
*Klor-Con 10	Potassium chloride	Electrolyte	
*Lanoxin	Digoxin	Cardiac glycoside	
*Lasix	Furosemide	Diuretic	
Lescol	Fluvastatin sodium	Antihyperlipidemic	
Levoxyl	Levothyroxine sodium	Thyroid preparation	
Lo/Ovral 28	Norgestrel, ethinyl estradiol	Oral contraceptive	
*Lodine	Etodolac	NSAID	
Loestrin FE 1.5/30	Ethinyl estradiol, norethindrone acetate	Oral contraceptive	
*Lopressor	Metoprolol tartrate	Antihypertensive (Beta-blocker)	
*Lorabid	Loracarbef	Antibiotic (Beta-lactam)	
Lorcet Plus	Hydrocodone bitartrate, acetaminophen	Narcotic and non-narcotic combo	(C-III)
*Lotensin	Benazepril hydrochloride	Antihypertensive	
Lotrisone	Clotrimazole and betamethasone dipropionate	Antifungal and anti-inflammatory	
*Lozol	Indapamide	Diuretic	
Macrobid	Nitrofurantoin monohydrated macrocrystals	Urinary germicide	
Medrol	Methylprednisolone	Glucocorticoid	
*Mevacor	Lovastatin	Antihyperlipidemic	

(continued on following page)

MOST COMMONLY PRESCRIBED BRAND-NAME MEDICATIONS *(continued from previous page)*

TRADE NAME	GENERIC	CLASSIFICATION	SCHEDULE
*Micro-K-10	Potassium chloride	Electrolyte	
*Micronase	Glyburide	Antidiabetic	
*Monopril	Fosinopril sodium	Antihypertensive	
*Motrin	Ibuprofen	NSAID	
*Naprosyn	Naproxen	NSAID, analgesic	
Nasacort	Triamcinolone acetonide	Corticosteroid	
Neomycin/Polymyxin B/Hydrocortisone	Cortisporin otic	Otic adrenocorticosteroid and antibiotic	
Nitro-Dur	Nitroglycerin transdermal infusion system	Coronary vasodilator, antianginal	
Nitrostat	Nitroglycerin (sublingual)	Coronary vasodilator, antianginal	
Nizoral Cream	Ketoconazole	Antifungal	
*Nizoral Tabs	Ketoconazole	Antifungal	
*Nolvadex	Tamoxifen	Antiestrogen	
Normodyne	Labetalol HCL	Antihypertensive	
*Norvasc	Amlodipine	Antihypertensive, antianginal	
Novolin 70/30	Human insulin	Insulin	
*Ogen	Estropipate	Estrogen	
Ortho-Cept 28	Desogestrel and ethinyl estradiol	Oral contraceptive	
Ortho-Novum 1/35-28	Norethindronel and ethinyl estradiol	Oral contraceptive	
Ortho-Novum 7/7/7-28	Norethindronel and ethinyl estradiol	Oral contraceptive	
Oruvail	Ketoprofen	NSAID	
*Paxil	Paroxetine hydrochloride	Antidepressant	
PCE	Erythromycin base	Antibiotic (Erythromycin)	
*Pepcid	Famotidine	Histamine H_2 receptor antagonist	

(continued on following page)

MOST COMMONLY PRESCRIBED BRAND-NAME MEDICATIONS *(continued from previous page)*

TRADE NAME	GENERIC	CLASSIFICATION	SCHEDULE
*Percocet	Oxycodone, acetaminophen	Narcotic and non-narcotic analgesic	(C-II)
Peridex	Chlorhexidine gluconate	Microbicidal oral rinse	
Phenergan	Promethazine hydrochloride	Antihistamine, antiemetic	
*Pravachol	Pravastatin sodium	Antihyperlipidemic	
Precose	Acarbose	Antidiabetic	
*Premarin (oral)	Conjugated estrogen	Estrogen replacement	
*Prilosec	Omeprazole	Antacid	
*Prinivil	Lisinopril	Antihypertensive	
*Procardia XL	Nifedipine	Antihypertensive, antianginal	
Propacet 100	Acetaminophen/propoxyphene	Narcotic and non-narcotic analgesic	(C-IV)
Propulsid	Cisapride	GI stimulant	
*Proscar	Finasteride	Androgen inhibitor	
*Proventil	Albuterol sulfate	Bronchodilator	
Proventil Inhalation Aerosol	Albuterol	Bronchodilator	
*Provera	Medroxyprogesterone acetate	Progestational hormone	
*Prozac	Fluoxetine hydrochloride	Antidepressant	
*Relafen	Nabumetone	NSAID	
*Restoril	Temazepam	Benzodiazepine hypnotic	(C-IV)
Retin A	Tretinoin	Antiacne drug	
*Ritalin	Methylphenidate hydrochloride	CNS stimulant	(C-II)
Roxicet	Oxycodone and acetaminophen	Narcotic and non-narcotic analgesic	(C-II)
*Seldane	Terfenadine	Antihistamine	
*Seldane D	Terfenadine, pseudoephedrine hydrochloride	Antihistamine and decongestant	

(continued on following page)

6

MOST COMMONLY PRESCRIBED BRAND-NAME MEDICATIONS *(continued from previous page)*

TRADE NAME	GENERIC	CLASSIFICATION	SCHEDULE
Serevent Inhalation Aerosol	Salmeterol xinafoate	Bronchodilator	
Sezone	Nefazone hydrochloride	Antidepressant	
Slo-bid	Theophylline	Antiasthmatic, bronchodilator	
Sumycin	Tetracycline hydrochloride	Antibiotic (Tetracycline)	
*Suprax	Cefixime	Cephalosporin (third-generation)	
*Synthroid	Levothyroxine sodium	Thyroid preparation	
*Tagamet	Cimetidine	Histamine H_2 receptor	
*Tegretol	Carbamazepine	Anticonvulsant	
*Tenex	Guanfacine hydrochloride	Antihypertensive	
*Tenormin	Atenolol	Antihypertensive (Beta-blocker)	
Terazol 7	Terconazole	Antifungal (vaginal)	
*Theo-Dur	Theophylline	Bronchodilator, antiasthmatic	
Timoptic	Timolol maleate	Ophthalmic agent	
*Toradol (oral)	Ketorolac tromethamine	NSAID	
*Trental	Pentoxifylline	Agent affecting the blood's viscosity	
Tri-Levlen (28)	Levonorgestrel and ethinyl estradiol	Oral contraceptive	
Trimox	Amoxicillin	Antibiotic (Penicillin)	
Triphasil-28	Levonorgestrel and ethinyl estradiol	Oral contraceptive	
Tylenol with codeine	Acetaminophen/codeine	Narcotic and non-narcotic analgesic	(C-III)
Ultram	Tramadol hydrochloride	Pain reliever	
*Valium	Diazepam	Antianxiety, anticonvulsant skeletal muscle relaxant	(C-IV)
Vancenase AQ	Beclomethasone dipropionate, monohydrate	Corticosteroid anti-inflammatory	
Vanceril	Beclomethasone dipropionate	Bronchodilator, glucocorticoid	

(continued on following page)

MOST COMMONLY PRESCRIBED BRAND-NAME MEDICATIONS *(continued from previous page)*

TRADE NAME	GENERIC	CLASSIFICATION	SCHEDULE
*Vasotec	Enalapril maleate	Angiotensin-converting enzyme inhibitor	
Veetids	Penicillin V Potassium	Antibiotic	
Ventolin Inhalation Aerosol	Albuterol	Bronchodilator	
Verelan	Verapamil hydrochloride	Ca-blocker, antianginal	
*Vicodin	Hydrocodone bitartrate, acetaminophen	Narcotic and non-narcotic analgesic	(C-III)
Vicodin ES	Hydrocodone bitartrate, acetaminophen	Narcotic and non-narcotic analgesic	(C-III)
*Voltaren	Diclofenac sodium	NSAID	
*Xanax	Alprazolam	Antianxiety	(C-IV)
*Zantac	Ranitidine hydrochloride	H₂ receptor antagonist	
*Zestril	Lisinopril	Antihypertensive, ACE inhibitor	
*Zithromax	Azithromycin	Antibiotic	
*Zocor	Simvastatin	Antihyperlipidemic	
*Zoloft	Sertraline hydrochloride	Antidepressant	
*Zovirax	Acyclovir	Antiviral, anti-infective	

6

MOST COMMONLY PRESCRIBED GENERIC MEDICATIONS

Medications indicated with an asterisk (*) appear in the drug insert.

GENERIC	BRAND EXAMPLES	CLASSIFICATION	SCHEDULE
*Acarbose	Precose	Antidiabetic	
*Acetaminophen and codeine	Tylenol with codeine	Narcotic and non-narcotic analgesic	(C-III)
Albuterol sulfate	Proventil	Bronchodilator	
Alendronate sodium	Fosamax	Antipostmenopausal osteoporosis	
Allopurinol	Zyloprim	Antigout	
*Alprazolam	Xanax	Antianxiety	(C-IV)
Amitriptyline HCL	Elavil	Antidepressant, tricyclic	
Amoxicillin trihydrate	Amoxicillin, Augmentin	Antibiotic (Penicillin)	
Ampicillin	Omnipen, Polycillin	Antibiotic (Penicillin)	
*Atenolol	Tenormin	Antihypertensive (Beta-adrenergic)	
Carisoprodol	Soma	Muscle relaxer	
*Cefaclor	Ceclor	Antibiotic	
Cephalexin	Keflex	Cephalosporin, anti-infective	
Cephalexin monohydrate	Keflex	Cephalosporin (first-generation)	
*Cimetidine	Tagamet	Antiulcer	
Clonidine HCL	Catapres	Antihypertensive	
*Cyclobenzaprine HCL	Flexeril	Skeletal muscle relaxant	
*Diazepam	Valium	Antianxiety	(C-IV)
Dicloxacillin sodium	Dynapen	Antibiotic	
Doxepin HCL	Adapin	Antidepressant	
Doxycycline hyclate	Vibramycin	Antibiotic (Tetracycline)	
Erythromycin base	E-Mycin	Antibiotic (Erythromycin)	

(continued on following page)

MOST COMMONLY PRESCRIBED GENERIC MEDICATIONS *(continued from previous page)*

GENERIC	BRAND EXAMPLES	CLASSIFICATION	SCHEDULE
Erythromycin ethylsuccinate	E.E.S.	Antibiotic (Erythromycin)	
Erythromycin stearate	Eramycin	Antibiotic (Erythromycin)	
Ferrous sulfate	Feosol	Antianemic (iron)	
Fiorinal with codeine	Fiorinal with codeine	Narcotic and non-narcotic analgesic	(C-III)
Folic Acid	Apo-Folic	Vitamin B complex	
*Furosemide	Lasix	Loop diuretic	
*Gemfibrozil	Lopid	Antihyperlipidemic	
*Glipizide	Glucotrol	Antidiabetic	
*Glyburide	Micronase	Oral hypoglycemic	
Guaifenesin	Robitussin	Expectorant	
Hydrochlorothiazide	Hydro DIURIL	Diuretic	
Hydrocodone with APAP	Lorcet Plus	Narcotic and non-narcotic analgesic	(C-III)
Hydrocortisone	Hydrocortone	Corticosteroid	
Hydroxyzine HCL	Atarax	Antianxiety	
Ibuprofen	Advil, Nuprin	NSAID	
imipramine HCL	Tofranil	Antidepressant	
*Isosorbide dinitrate	Isordil	Coronary vasodilator, antianginal	
Lithium carbonate	LITHOBID	Antipsychotic agent	
*Lorazepam	Ativan	Antianxiety	(C-IV)
*Losartan potassium	Cozaar	Antihypertensive	
Meclizine HCL	Antivert	Antiemetic, antihistamine, antimotion sickness	
*Medroxyprogesterone acetate	Provera	Progesterone	
*Metformin	Glucophage	Antidiabetic	

(continued on following page)

MOST COMMONLY PRESCRIBED GENERIC MEDICATIONS *(continued from previous page)*

GENERIC	BRAND EXAMPLES	CLASSIFICATION	SCHEDULE
*Methylphenidate HCL	Ritalin	CNS stimulant	(C-II)
*Metoprolol tartrate	Lopressor	Antihypertensive	
Metronidazole HCL	Flagyl	Systemic trichomonacide, amebicide, antibiotic	
*Naproxen	Naprosyn	NSAID	
*Naproxen sodium	Anaprox	NSAID, analgesic	
*Nefazadone HCL	Serone	Antidepressant	
Nitroglycerine	Nitrostat	Coronary vasodilator, antianginal	
*Nortriptyline HCL	Pamelor	Antidepressant, tricyclic	
Nystatin	Mycostatin	Antibiotic, antifungal	
*Penicillin VK	Pen-Vee K	Antibiotic	
Phenobarbital	Solfoton	Sedative, anticonvulsant	(C-IV)
Potassium chloride	K-Lyte	Electrolyte	
*Prednisone	Deltasone	Corticosteroid	
Promethazine HCL	Phenergan	Antihistamine, antiemetic	
Propoxyphene napsylate	Darvocet-N 100	Narcotic and non-narcotic analgesic	(C-IV)
*Temazepam	Restoril	Hypnotic	(C-III)
Tetracycline HCL	Panmycin, Sumycin	Antibiotic (Tetracycline)	
Trazodone HCL	Desyrel	Antidepressant	
Triamcinolone	Aristocort, Kenacort	Corticosteroid	
*Triamterene and HCTZ	Dyazide	Diuretic, antihypertensive	
*Trimethoprim and sulfamethoxazole	Bactrim, Septra	Antibacterial	
*Verapamil HCL	Calan SR	Antianginal, antihypertensive	

(continued on following page)

MOST COMMONLY PRESCRIBED GENERIC MEDICATIONS *(continued from previous page)*

GENERIC	BRAND EXAMPLES	CLASSIFICATION	SCHEDULE

6

Over-the-Counter
Medication Instructions

The following chart lists some of the more commonly used OTC (over-the-counter) medications. The chart can be used in a variety of ways. It can help the assistant spell an OTC medication and can also be helpful in telephone triaging.

The assessment charts sometimes refer to OTC medications. The third column might read OTC, followed by a category, i.e., analgesic. The chart will provide the assistant with a few of the more common drugs that are available over-the-counter.

Before using the following chart, it is important for the assistant to confer with the physician to see if he or she agrees with the medications that are listed on the chart. Extra space is provided that will allow the assistant to personalize the chart with some of the more common OTC drugs that are more routinely recommended by the physician.

If the physician prefers to personalize charts for specific needs of the practice, Section 12 contains two blank OTC medication forms: one a pediatric form, the other an adult form. Remember that these drugs must be preapproved by the physician before being offered to the patient. (Many physicians will want to do this on a case-by-case basis.) This will help alleviate possible legal problems.

How to Use the OTC Charts

1. When using the assessment charts in Section 3 and the telephone triage column instructs the assistant to suggest an OTC medication, turn to page 118, OTC Medication Questions.

2. Ask the patient each of the questions that appears on the OTC question form (page 118).

3. If the patient answers yes to any of those questions, ask the physician what medication the patient should be able to take.

4. If the patient answers no to all of the questions, refer to the form labeled Leading OTC Medications (page 119), if this is the form the physician wants you to use.

5. If the physician prefers using the personalized OTC charts in Section 12, turn to the adult or pediatric chart as necessary.

6. Once the appropriate chart has been located, scan the page until the drug classification that was suggested on the assessment chart, e.g., OTC decongestant, is found.

7. Suggest one of the medications listed under the appropriate category.

8. Refer back to the original assessment chart in Section 3 if the assessment questions have not been completed.

9. Refer back to the telephone triage chart in Section 2 if the assessment questions have been completed.

Over-the-Counter
Medication Questions

Before providing any over-the-counter medication suggestions, the assistant should read the OTC instructions.

Once the assistant has read the OTC instructions, the patient should be asked the following questions:

1. Do you have any drug allergies?

2. Do you currently take any prescribed medications? List them.

3. Is the medication being suggested available or accessible to you?

4. Have you taken any OTC medications or tried any other home remedies for your current condition? (When was your last dose, and how much did you take? Did you receive any relief?)

5. Do you have any other diseases that the physician should be aware of?

If the patient answers yes to any of the above questions, check with the physician before making any suggestions.

The assistant should make sure the physician has preapproved the OTC chart and that the exact protocol on the assessment form is being followed before suggesting any OTC medications.

LEADING OVER-THE-COUNTER MEDICATIONS

ADULT COUGH MEDICATIONS
Robitussin-DM, Delsym

ADULT COLD REMEDIES
Drixoral, Comtrex, Tavist D, Nyquil
Robitussin-CF, Vicks Formula 44 M

MULTISYMPTOM/FLU REMEDIES
Theraflu, Comtrex

NASAL DECONGESTANT
Afrin (Liq/Spray), Neo-Synephrine (Liq/Spray)
Sudafed (Tabs), Drixoral (Tabs)

SORE THROAT REMEDIES
Chloraseptic, Cepastat, Sucrets

HAY FEVER/ALLERGY
Benadryl, Dimetapp, Dimetapp Elixir, Tavist D
Chlor-Trimenton

SINUS REMEDIES
Sinutab, Sudafed, Tylenol Sinus

ADULT ANALGESICS
Advil, Tylenol Extra Strength, Motrin B, Excedrin

EXTERNAL ANALGESICS
Myoflex, Flexall 454, Aspercreme, Ben-Gay

SLEEPING AIDS
Unisom, Benadryl, Sominex, Nyquil

ANTACIDS
Mylanta, Mylanta II, Maalox, Tums

ANTIFLATULENT
Mylicon, Gas X

ANTIDIARRHEALS
Imodium A-D, Kaopectate

FIBER LAXATIVE/SUPPLEMENT
Metamucil, FiberCon, Citrucel, Perdiem

SOFTENER/STIMULANT LAXATIVE
Colace, Dulcolax, Ex-Lax

HEMORRHOIDAL PREPARATIONS
Preparation H, Anusol-HC

VAGINAL ANTIFUNGALS
Monistat 7, Gyne-Lotrimin

VAGINAL MOISTURIZER
Replens, K-Y Jelly, Gyne-Moistrin

(continued on following page)

LEADING OVER-THE-COUNTER MEDICATIONS *(continued from previous page)*

JOCK ITCH PREPARATIONS
Tinactin, Lotrimin, Micatin, Cruex

ANTI-ITCH/RASH PREPARATIONS
Cortizone, Cortaid

POISON IVY-OAK PREPARATIONS
Caladryl, Ivy Dry

ATHLETE'S FOOT PREPARATIONS
Lotrimin AF, Tinnactin, Micatin

FOOT CARE PRODUCTS
Dr. Scholl, Johnson's Foot Soap

EMOLLIENTS AND PROTECTIVE SKIN PRODUCTS
Eucerin, Lubriderm

WOUND CARE PRODUCTS
Neosporin, Triple Antibiotic Ointment

CANKER SORE PRODUCTS
Orabase B, Zilactin, Tanac

DENTAL MOUTHWASH
Listerine, Scope, Cepacol

EYE DROPS
Visine, Murine

ANTILOUSE PREPARATIONS
Nix, Rid, A-200

DIET AIDS
Dexatrim, Slim Fast, Acutrim

PEDIATRIC COLD PREPARATIONS
Dimetapp Liquid, Pediacare, Triaminic

PEDIATRIC COUGH PREPARATIONS
Robitussin Pediatric, Naldecon-DX, Robitussin DM

PEDIATRIC ANALGESIC
Tylenol Drops

ANTIOXIDENT VITAMINS AND MINERALS
Protegra, Centrum

CALCIUM SUPPLEMENTS
Os-Cal, Citracal

BLOOD GLUCOSE METERS
One Touch, One Touch II, Glucometer III

OVULATION PREDICTORS
First Response, Clear Plan Easy, OvuQuick

PREGNANCY TEST KIT
e.p.t., Clearblue Easy, First Response, Fact Plus

(continued on following page)

LEADING OVER-THE-COUNTER MEDICATIONS *(continued from previous page)*

LATEST/FUTURE OTC DRUGS

The following drug list is currently being considered for nonprescription status. By the time this book is published it is likely that many will already be approved for OTC use. Check with your local pharmacy for the latest updates.

Topical Erythromycin (Antiacne)	Nicorette (Antismoking)	Claritin (Antihistamine, without drowsiness)
Cromolyn (Asthma, Allergies)	Axid (Antiulcer)	Carafate (Antiulcer)
Zantac (Antiulcer)	Ketoprofen (NSAID, Analgesic)	Piroxicam (NSAID, Analgesic)
Aleve (NSAID, Analgesic)		

Physician's Approval: _____

Dosage Calculations and Formulas

Pediatric Dosage Calculations

It is recommended that when calculating the medication dosage for a child that the method of dosage per kilogram of body weight or body-surface area be used for accuracy.

Pediatric dose = child's body WT (kg) x mg of drug/kg

Example: 100 mg/kg/day dose medication

child's weight is 10 kg

X mg is unknown dosage

100 mg: 1 kg :: X mg: 10 kg

1 kg $\times$ X mg = 100 mg $\times$ 10 kg

$X = 100$ mg $\times$ 10 kg

$X = 1000$ mg

Using the body surface area nomogram (see next page) to determine the BSA (body surface area) of the child, the pediatric dose may be figured as:

child's dose = m^2 (child's BSA) $\times$ (drug dose) mg

Example: child's dose = $.8^2 \times 500$ mg

child's dose = $.64 \times 500$ mg

child's dose = 320 mg

When the adult dose is known, a child's dose may be figured as:

$$\text{child's dose} = \frac{\text{child's BSA } m^2}{\text{average adult BSA}} \times \text{average adult dose}$$
$$(1.7 \text{ m}^2)$$

Example: child's dose = $\dfrac{1.6^2}{1.7^2} \times 250$ mg

$$\text{child's dose} = \frac{2.56}{2.89} \times 250 \text{ mg}$$

$$\text{child's dose} = \frac{640}{2.89}$$

$$\text{child's dose} = 221.45 \text{ mg}$$

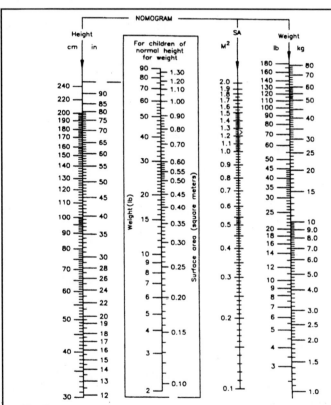

NOMOGRAM

Directions:

1. Determine height on left vertical column.
2. Determine weight on right vertical column.
3. Draw a straight line to connect the height and weight.
4. Where the line intersects on the surface area is the derived body surface area (m^2).

From Mosby's Medical, Nursing, & Allied Health Dictionary, 4th ed. (St. Louis: Mosby-YearBook, Inc., 1994.)

Fried's Rule—used for a child under 12 months of age:

$$\frac{\text{child's age in months}}{150 \text{ months}} \times \text{average adult dose} = \text{child's dose}$$

(150 months is the age when an adult dose would be appropriate)

Example: $\dfrac{5 \text{ months}}{150 \text{ months}} \times 250 \text{ mg} = \dfrac{1250}{150} = 8.33 \text{ mg}$ (child's dose)

Clark's Rule—used for a child over 2 years of age:

$$\frac{\text{child's weight (lbs)}}{150 \text{ lbs}} \times \text{average adult dose} = \text{child's dose}$$

Example: $\dfrac{50 \text{ lbs}}{150 \text{ lbs}} \times 500 \text{ mg} = \text{child's dose}$

$$\frac{25000}{150} = \text{child's dose}$$

$$166.66 \text{ mg} = \text{child's dose}$$

Young's Rule—used for a child between the ages of 2 to 12 years of age:

$$\frac{\text{child's age in years}}{\text{child's age in years} + 12} \times \text{average adult dose} = \text{child's dose}$$

Example: $\dfrac{10}{10+12} \times 250 = \text{child's dose}$

$$\frac{2500}{22} = \text{child's dose}$$

$$113.63 = \text{child's dose}$$

Adult Dosage Calculations

$$\frac{\text{Amount desired}}{\text{Amount available}} \times \text{quantity} = X$$

If the physician ordered 30 mg of Lasix and the vial reads 60mg/1 cc of medication, how much should the patient have been given?

$$\frac{30 \text{ mg}}{60 \text{ mg}} \quad 1 \text{ cc} = 1/2 \text{ or } 0.5 \text{ cc}$$

Body Mass Index

To find the body mass index (BMI), place weight over height squared and multiply by 705.

$$\text{BMI} = \frac{\text{WT}}{\text{HT}^2} \times 705$$

Example: WT = 167 lbs; HT = 67"

HT squared = 4489

$$\text{BMI} = \frac{167}{4489} \times 705$$

$$\text{BMI} = \frac{117735}{4489}$$

BMI = 26.22

Ratio and Proportion

Example:

6 is to 30 as x is to 400

$$30 x = 2400$$

$$x = 80$$

Converting Measurements

LENGTH	Centimeters	Inches	Feet
1 centimeter	1.000	0.394	0.0328
1 inch	2.54	1.000	0.0833
1 foot	30.48	12.000	1.000
1 yard	91.4	36.00	3.00
1 meter	100.00	39.40	3.28

VOLUMES	Cubic Centimeters	Fluid Drams	Fluid Ounces	Quarts	Liters
1 cubic centimeter	1.00	0.270	0.033	0.0010	0.0010
1 fluid dram	3.70	1.00	0.125	0.0090	0.0037
1 cubic inch	16.39	4.43	0.554	0.0173	0.0163
1 fluid ounce	29.6	8.00	1.000	0.0312	0.0296
1 quart	946.0	255.0	32.0	1.00	0.946
1 liter	1000.0	270.0	33.80	1.056	1.000

WEIGHTS	Grains	Grams	Apothecary Ounces	Pounds
1 grain (gr)	1.000	0.064	0.002	0.0001
1 gram (gm)	15.43	1.000	0.032	0.0022
1 apothecary ounce	480.00	31.1	1.000	0.0685
1 pound	7000.00	454.0	14.58	1.000
1 kilogram	15432.0	1000.0	32.15	2.205

Rules for Converting from One System to Another

Lengths

Inches to centimeters—multiply by 2.54

Feet to centimeters—multiply by 30.48

Centimeters to inches—divide by 2.54

Centimeters to feet—divide by 30.48

Volumes

Grains to grams—divide by 15

Drams to cubic centimeters—multiply by 4

Ounces to cubic centimeters—multiply by 30

Minims to cubic millimeters—multiply by 63

Minims to cubic centimeters—multiply by 0.06

Cubic millimeters to minims—divide by 63

Cubic centimeters to minims—multiply by 16

Cubic centimeters to fluid ounces—divide by 30

Liters to pints—divide by 2.1

Weights

Milligrams to grains—multiply by 0.0154

Grams to grains—multiply by 15

Grams to drams—multiply by 0.257

Grams to ounces—multiply by 0.0311

Pounds to kilograms—divide by 2.2

Kilograms to pounds—multiply by 2.2

Temperature

To convert Fahrenheit to Celsius: Multiply Centigrade degrees by 9/5 and add 32:

C = (F − 32) × 5/9 or 37° C = 98.6° F − 32 = 66.6 × 5/9 (333/9)

Example: 38 = (F −32) × 5/9

  C = (91.4 − 32) × 5/9

  C = 59.4 × 5/9

  C = 6.6 × 5

  C = 33

To convert Celsius to Fahrenheit: Subtract 32 from the Fahrenheit degrees and multiply by 5/9:

F = (C × 9/5) + 32 or 98.6° F = 37° C × 9/5 (333/5) = 66.6 + 32

Example: F = (38 × 9/5) + 32

  $F = \dfrac{342}{5} + 32$

  F = 68.4 + 32

  F = 100.4

Household Measures and Weights

1 teaspoon	= 1/6 fluid ounce or 1 dram
3 teaspoons	= 1 tablespoon
1 dessert spoon	= 1/3 fluid ounce or 2 drams
1 tablespoon	= 1/2 fluid ounce or 3 drams
4 tablespoons	= 1 wine glass or 1/2 gill
16 tablespoons (liq)	= 1 cup
12 tablespoons (dry)	= 1 cup
1 cup	= 8 fluid ounces
1 tumbler or glass	= 8 fluid ounces or 1/2 pint
1 wine glass	= 2 fluid ounces
16 fluid ounces	= 1 pound
4 gills	= 1 pound
1 pint	= 1 pound

Traditional Time and 24-Hour Time

In the 24-hour day, the exact time must be observed to accurately document patient care. Recording the exact time can be critical in the course of medical conditions, procedures, and treatments. Differentiating between day and night also is necessary. The following information offers what is commonly known as 24-hour time or military time, and standardized or traditional time.

Beginning with midnight, time is read in the traditional or standard form as 12:00 AM. At 1:00 (one) AM standard/traditional time, military time is 100 hours (said "O" 100 hours) and so on to 0900 ("O" nine hundred hours), or 900 hours. At noon, traditional/standard time is read as 12:00 PM; military or 24-hour time is 1200 hours.

For all PM hours, time is read by adding 12 to the number of each hour, i.e., 1:00 PM is 1300 hours. (1:00 plus 12 is 1300). A list of the times for each system follows.

Standard/traditional	24 hour/military
12:00 AM (midnight)	0 (zero) hundred hours (or 2400 hours)
1:00 AM	0100 (one hundred) hours
2:00 AM	0200 (two hundred) hours
3:00 AM	0300 (three hundred) hours
4:00 AM	0400 (four hundred) hours
5:00 AM	0500 (five hundred) hours
6:00 AM	0600 (six hundred) hours
7:00 AM	0700 (seven hundred) hours
8:00 AM	0800 (eight hundred) hours
9:00 AM	0900 (nine hundred) hours
10:00 AM	1000 (ten hundred) hours
11:00 AM	1100 (eleven hundred) hours
12:00 PM (noon)	1200 (twelve hundred) hours
1:00 PM	1300 (thirteen hundred) hours
2:00 PM	1400 (fourteen hundred) hours
3:00 PM	1500 (fifteen hundred) hours
4:00 PM	1600 (sixteen hundred) hours
5:00 PM	1700 (seventeen hundred) hours
6:00 PM	1800 (eighteen hundred) hours

Standard/traditional	24 hour/military
7:00 PM	1900 (nineteen hundred) hours
8:00 PM	2000 (twenty hundred) hours
9:00 PM	2100 (twenty-one hundred) hours
10:00 PM	2200 (twenty-two hundred) hours
11:00 PM	2300 (twenty-three hundred) hours

SECTION

7

INSTRUMENTS

Introduction

I n this section are illustrations of instruments labeled with their correct names. The groups are comprised of instruments that are used for particular body systems or that are related because of their use, i.e., eye, ear, nose, and throat instruments are grouped together for quick reference, as are surgical instruments.

For efficient communication, it is important that the assistant be able to identify instruments by their proper given names.

Proper care and sterilization of instruments is vital for their longevity. Since these items are costly, it is important to treat instruments with care and respect. Instructions regarding the proper methods to clean and sterilize each instrument are included from the manufacturer. The assistant must pay close attention to this detail as each instrument is unwrapped from its packaging. Each instrument should be inspected for any flaws or malfunctions upon its arrival and thereafter following each use, when it is being sanitized and prepared for sterilization. An instrument should be used solely for the purpose for which it was made. The assistant should always wear latex gloves (double glove, PRN) for protection against microorganisms. All instruments should be properly sanitized after use by employing the following steps:

1. Rinse in cool water to remove excess secretions.

2. Soak in a detergent and warm water solution for at least twenty minutes to loosen and lift away any material that could have adhered to the metal during use.

   a. Solution should be of a neutral pH (near 7.0).

3. Scrub instruments with a medium-soft brush to loosen particles from the surface; include crevices and hinges.

   a. Use a fresh solution of comfortably hot water and detergent.

4. Rinse each instrument well to remove all traces of detergent residue.

   a. Inspect each instrument for any flaws, snags, chips, sprung hinges, or any other malfunction.

   b. Report nonusable instruments to the supervisor/employer for replacement.

5. Place instruments with hinges and/or moving parts in a lubricating solution before sterilizing.

6. Wrap instruments and appropriately date, label, and initial them.

7. Sterilize/autoclave for the required amount of time as appropriate for packaged material.

The assistant should never place an instrument that is not of top-functioning quality into a chemical disinfecting solution or as part of a packet to be autoclaved. The possibility of a malfunctioning instrument being used on patients could be detrimental to the patients themselves, coworkers, the physician, or the assistant. Remove the instrument at once to eliminate any possibility of injury. A written documentation should be made and a replacement ordered for the faulty instrument. The employer's policy should be followed for proper protocol. The date and signature should be on the report—safety comes first for all concerned!

Illustrations of Instruments

Curved Surgical Scissors

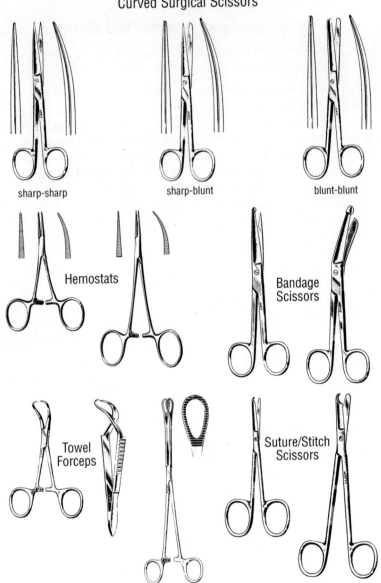

sharp-sharp   sharp-blunt   blunt-blunt

Hemostats

Bandage Scissors

Towel Forceps

Suture/Stitch Scissors

Sponge-holding Forceps

(Courtesy of J. Jamner Surgical Instruments, Inc.)

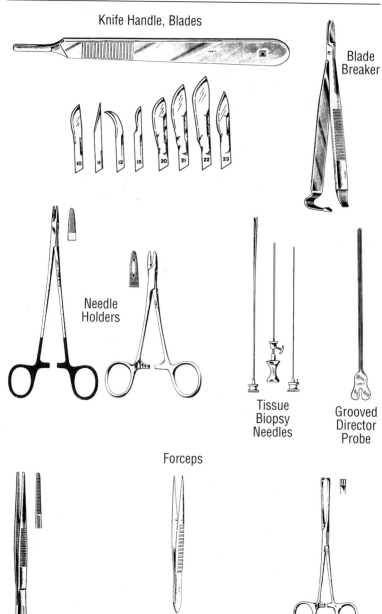

Knife Handle, Blades

Blade Breaker

Needle Holders

Tissue Biopsy Needles

Grooved Director Probe

Forceps

thumb

splinter

tissue

(Courtesy of J. Jamner Surgical Instruments, Inc.)

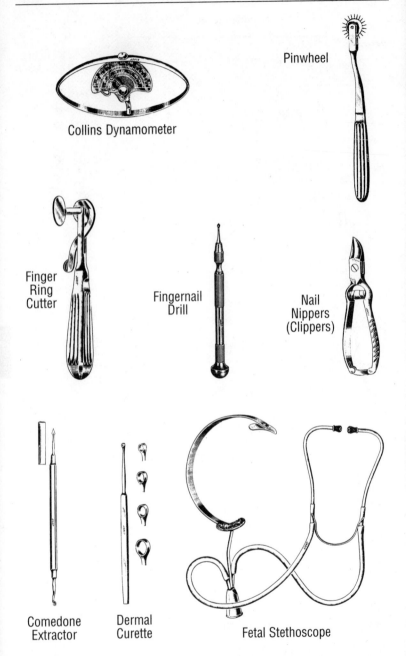

Pinwheel

Collins Dynamometer

Finger
Ring
Cutter

Fingernail
Drill

Nail
Nippers
(Clippers)

Comedone
Extractor

Dermal
Curette

Fetal Stethoscope

(Courtesy of J. Jamner Surgical Instruments, Inc.)

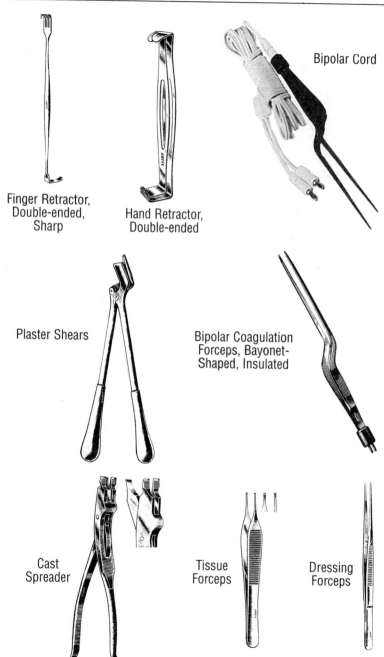

Finger Retractor,
Double-ended,
Sharp

Hand Retractor,
Double-ended

Bipolar Cord

Plaster Shears

Bipolar Coagulation
Forceps, Bayonet-
Shaped, Insulated

Cast
Spreader

Tissue
Forceps

Dressing
Forceps

(Courtesy of J. Jamner Surgical Instruments, Inc.)

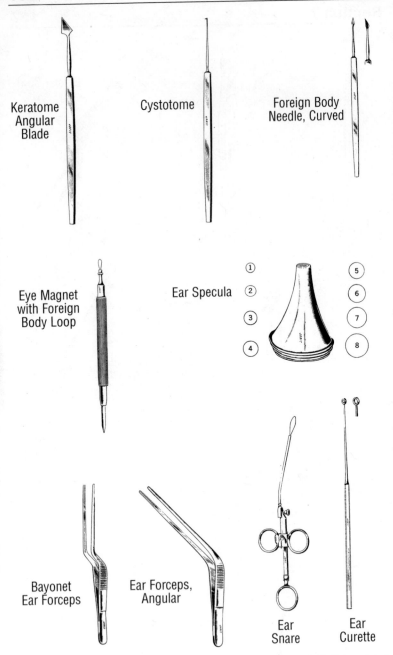

Keratome Angular Blade

Cystotome

Foreign Body Needle, Curved

Eye Magnet with Foreign Body Loop

Ear Specula

① ② ③ ④ ⑤ ⑥ ⑦ ⑧

Bayonet Ear Forceps

Ear Forceps, Angular

Ear Snare

Ear Curette

(Courtesy of J. Jamner Surgical Instruments, Inc.)

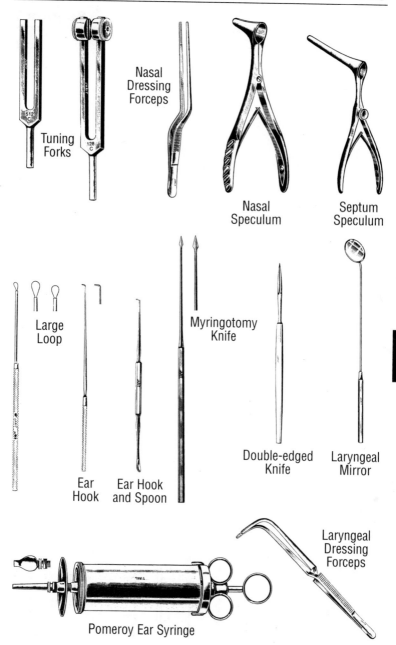

Tuning Forks

Nasal Dressing Forceps

Nasal Speculum

Septum Speculum

Large Loop

Ear Hook

Ear Hook and Spoon

Myringotomy Knife

Double-edged Knife

Laryngeal Mirror

Pomeroy Ear Syringe

Laryngeal Dressing Forceps

(Courtesy of J. Jamner Surgical Instruments, Inc.)

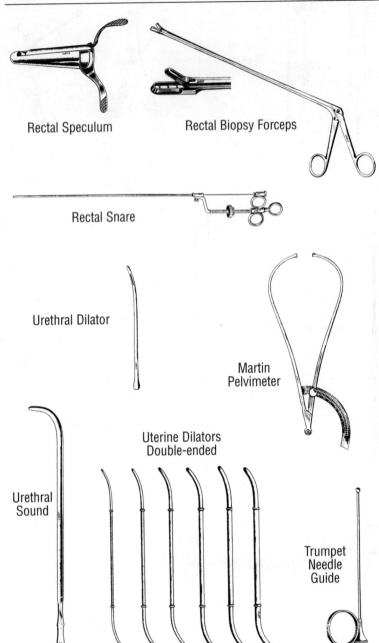

Rectal Speculum

Rectal Biopsy Forceps

Rectal Snare

Urethral Dilator

Martin Pelvimeter

Uterine Dilators Double-ended

Urethral Sound

Trumpet Needle Guide

(Courtesy of J. Jamner Surgical Instruments, Inc.)

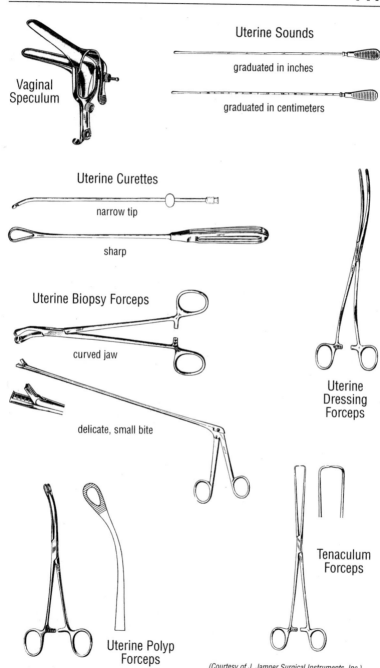

Vaginal Speculum

Uterine Sounds

graduated in inches

graduated in centimeters

Uterine Curettes

narrow tip

sharp

Uterine Biopsy Forceps

curved jaw

delicate, small bite

Uterine Dressing Forceps

Uterine Polyp Forceps

Tenaculum Forceps

(Courtesy of J. Jamner Surgical Instruments, Inc.)

SECTION

8.

TRAY SETUPS

Introduction

The following section lists many of the common tray setups that are used in a family practice setting. Each of the forms has extra lines to add any additional items that may not appear on the form but that are routinely used in the office.

There also is a place to make other modifications on each of the charts, as well as a place for the physician's approval.

COMPLETE PHYSICAL EXAM

TRAY SETUP

Stethoscope
Sphygmomanometer
Penlight
Guaiac test developer
Flexible tape measure
Lubricant

Guaiac blood test
Urine specimen container
Nasal speculum
Tuning fork
Ear speculum/curette
Latex gloves

Percussion hammer
Tongue depressor
Ophthalmoscope
Otoscope

Other supplies:
_____
_____
_____
_____

TIPS

1. Explain procedure to patient.
2. Give patient gown and drape sheet.
3. Check to see if doctor would like any diagnostic testing, i.e., Xrays, lab work, EKG, etc.

4. Do not allow patient to have anything to eat or drink until after the exam.
5. Check batteries of scope handle for proper functioning.
6. Fill out lab requisition forms prior to exam. (Obtain physician's order first.)

Any Modifications:
_____
_____
_____
_____
_____

Physician's Approval: _____

8

CYST REMOVAL TRAY

WHAT'S ON THE TRAY	WHAT'S OFF TO THE SIDE	TIPS
Scalpel handle and blade	Biohazard container	Try to position the patient in a comfortable position
Needle holder	Sterile gloves	Lighting needs to be positioned directly over cyst (if possible)
Dissecting scissors	Alcohol	Set supplies in order of use
Operating scissors	Cotton balls	Be available to assist physician throughout the procedure
Tissue forceps	Local anesthetic	Try to reassure patient throughout the procedure
Hemostatic forceps	Sterile gauze bandaging	Watch patient's expression (if uncomfortable, alert doctor)
Thumb forceps	Surgical tape	Have specimen container ready for physician
Suture material	Lab requisition form	Be ready to apply sterile dressing following procedure
Sterile containers (2)	Specimen container (lab)	Have any prescriptions ready for patient
Cotton-tipped applicators	Sterile syringe and needle	Have any home care instructions ready for patient
Sterile 4×4s	Antiseptic solution	Assist patient to the receptionist to schedule a follow-up visit
Fenestrated drape		

Any Modifications:

_____

_____

_____

_____

Physician's Approval: _____

EYE, EAR, NOSE AND THROAT TRAY

INSTRUMENTS AND SUPPLIES

Ophthalmoscope	Tongue depressor	. Other supplies:
Otoscope with ear speculum	Nasal speculum	
Tuning fork	Cotton-tipped applicators	
Penlight	Tissues	
	Latex gloves	
	Appropriate cultures	
	Appropriate medications	
	Drape-lined tray	

TIPS

1. Set supplies up in order of use.
2. Explain what to expect from the exam to help the patient relax.
3. Assist patient with removing/replacing glasses, hearing aids, etc., and on and off exam table.
4. Assist with or obtain cultures as directed by physician.
5. Drape patient according to procedure that is being done. (Try to keep patient dry.)
6. Be available to turn lights on and off as needed during the exam, according to the physician's preference.
7. Label cultures and complete lab request forms. Enter appropriate information into log books.

Any Modifications: _____

_____

_____

_____

_____

Physician's Approval: _____

ELECTROSURGICAL TRAY

ITEMS NECESSARY

Hyfrecator (cautery unit)

Cautery needle

Grounding plate

Biohazard bag/container

Operating scissors

Routine procedure to remove warts, moles, and lesions

Tissue forceps

Latex gloves (sterile)

Sterile gauze pads (4×4s)

Betadine

Biopsy container

Other supplies:

_____

_____

_____

_____

Any Modifications:

_____

_____

_____

_____

_____

Physician's Approval: _____

INCISION AND DRAINAGE TRAY

ITEMS PLACED DIRECTLY ONTO THE FIELD	ITEMS PLACED OFF TO THE SIDE OF THE STERILE FIELD
Scalpel blade (usually #15, check with physician first)	Sterile gloves (a pair for the physician and in some cases a pair for the assistant)
Scalpel handle (some of the disposable packs come with both the handle and the blade)	Packing material (usually Iodoform Gauze, or Sterile Kling for packing)
Hemostatic forceps	Penrose drain
Dissecting scissors	Antiseptic solution (Pour the solution directly into the sterile container that is already on the tray.)
Thumb forceps	Dressing material
Tissue forceps	Surgical tape
Operating scissors	Alcohol/cotton (to cleanse anesthetic vial)
Needle/syringe	Anesthetic (Check to see what type, what strength, and if it should be with or without epinephrine.)
Cotton-tipped applicators	Sterile gauze squares (usually 4×4s or 3×3s)
Fenestrated drape	Biohazard bag/container
Sterile drape	Prescriptions ready (antibiotic/pain killer) Get direct order from the physician first.
Sterile containers (2)	Home Care Instruction Sheet should be attached to the chart to give to the patient following the procedure.
	Patient's chart

The assistant is usually considered nonsterile until the end of the procedure. He or she may then have to apply a sterile bandage to the area and must be available to retrieve any extras the physician may need during the procedure. Check on the patient several times during the procedure. If you notice that the patient is uncomfortable, notify the physician right away.

As always, make sure the patient reads, understands, and signs the consent form prior to the procedure being performed.

(continued on following page)

8

INCISION AND DRAINAGE TRAY *(continued from previous page)*

Any Modifications: _____

_____

_____

_____

_____

_____

Physician's Approval: _____

INJECTING A JOINT TRAY

ITEMS NECESSARY

Sterile latex gloves

Antiseptic solution (i.e., Betadine)

Cotton-tipped applicators

Gauze squares (usually 4×4s)

Anesthetic (get specific order from physician)

Medication (get specific order from physician,

i.e., Depomedrol)

Needle (check with physician for exact size)

Band-Aid®

Other supplies:

_____

_____

_____

Any Modifications:

_____

_____

_____

_____

Physician's Approval:_____

LACERATION/SUTURE TRAY

LACERATION TRAY

ITEMS TO BE PLACED DIRECTLY ON THE STERILE FIELD

Needle driver/holder

Appropriate suture material

Hemostats

Surgical scissors

Tissue forceps

Transfer forceps

Gauze squares

Needle/syringe

Cotton-tipped applicators

Fenestrated drape

Solution containers (usually two)

ITEMS TO BE PLACED OFF TO THE SIDE

Bandage scissors

Biohazard bag/container

Bandaging material/antiseptic cream

Tape

Sterile irrigation solution, i.e., saline

Antiseptic swabs/solution, i.e., Betadine

Alcohol/cotton balls

Sterile latex gloves (physician and assistant)

Ordered anesthetic

Mayo stand/sterile drape

PPE (face shield/mask/gown)

Patient's chart

Tetanus immunization (when necessary)

Any Modifications:

Physician's Approval:

PAP AND PELVIC TRAY

PAP TRAY

WHAT'S ON THE TRAY	WHAT'S OFF TO THE SIDE	HELPFUL TIPS
Vaginal speculum	Patient drape	Ask patient to empty bladder.
		(Obtain urine sample if patient is symptomatic.)
Two or more frosted slides	Patient gown	Explain exam to patient.
Lubricant (i.e., KY Jelly)	Patient's chart	Explain how to put on gown/drape.
Endocervical brush	Gooseneck lamp	Answer patient's questions and relieve anxiety.
Cervical scraper	Mayo stand (not for every office)	Discuss when to return/call for report.
Container to hold slides	Tissues/towel	Be sure that speculum is warmed prior to insertion.
Fixative	Gloves	
Cotton-tipped applicators		
Cultures (if instructed)		

PELVIC TRAY

WHAT'S ON THE TRAY	WHAT'S OFF TO THE SIDE	HELPFUL TIPS
Vaginal speculum	Patient drape	Remember to advise patient to empty bladder.
		(Check to see if physician wants a specimen.)
Water-soluble lubricant	Patient gown	Give patient tips on how to relax, i.e., breathe in through nose and out through mouth.
Cotton-tipped applicators	Gooseneck lamp	Explain to patient what articles of clothing need to be removed and where to place them.

(continued on following page)

PAP AND PELVIC TRAY *(continued from previous page)*

PELVIC TRAY

WHAT'S ON THE TRAY	WHAT'S OFF TO THE SIDE	HELPFUL TIPS
Gauze squares	Mayo stand	Assist patient to and from table for safety
Appropriate cultures, tubes, glass slides, ayer blade, uterine sound, uterine dressing forceps (when indicated by physician)	Patient's chart	Discuss when patient can call for lab results (give code number when applicable).
	Gloves	Make sure speculum is warmed before insertion.
	Cytology request form	

Any Modifications:

_____

_____

_____

_____

Physician's Approval: _____

RECTAL EXAM TRAY

ITEMS NECESSARY

Latex gloves

Water-soluble lubricant (i.e., KY Jelly)

Proctoscope/anoscope

Cotton-tipped applicators

Tissues

Guaiac test/developer

Drape sheet

Biohazard bag

Other supplies:

_____

_____

_____

Usually done on patients who are experiencing rectal bleeding or pain. Protecting the patient's modesty is crucial!

Any Modifications: _____

_____

_____

_____

_____

Physician's Approval: _____

SIGMOIDOSCOPY TRAY

TRAY SETUP

Latex gloves
Lubricant
Sigmoidoscope
Long cotton-tip swabs
Drape sheet

Suction machine (water should be at
room temperature.)
Tissues
Biopsy forceps
Specimen container

Lab request form
Tissue forceps
Patient's chart

Other supplies:
_____
_____
_____
_____

TIPS

1. Confirm appointment with patient the day before the procedure.
2. Check to make sure the equipment is working the day before the procedure is scheduled so the patient can be forewarned should there be a problem.
3. Explain the procedure to the patient prior to the exam.

4. Have patient sign consent form prior to procedure.
5. Take measures to protect the patient's modesty.
6. Comfort the patient as much as possible during the exam.
7. Check with the physician prior to the exam to see if he or she would like to have any medications available during exam, e.g., Levsin.

Any Modifications:
_____
_____
_____
_____
_____

Physician's Approval: _____

SUTURE REMOVAL TRAY

ITEMS TO BE PLACED DIRECTLY ONTO FIELD

Gauze squares

Cotton-tip applicators

Suture removal scissors

Thumb forceps

ITEMS TO BE PLACED OFF TO THE SIDE

Latex gloves (sterile)

Bandaging supplies/antiseptic ointment (Band-Aid®)

Basin/irrigation solution, i.e., peroxide, saline

Biohazard bag

Patient's chart

Suture Removal Tips:

1. Use hydrogen peroxide or warm soapy water if sutures are stuck to the skin or bandage.

2. Clip suture as close to the skin as possible, without cutting the patient.

3. Always pull the suture toward the wound/incision.

Any Modifications:

Physician's Approval:_____

8

SECTION

9

PROCEDURES, TIPS, AND FACTS

Introduction

The procedure section of the book lists the most common procedures that are done in a general practice setting. The procedure charts do not list the specific steps for each procedure, but instead list the supplies necessary to perform the procedure. Valuable facts and troubleshooting tips are also offered.

Any lab tests considered moderate complexity or high complexity tests were intentionally omitted, as were many diagnostic tests and procedures that involved some kind of automation, due to the fact that several styles of units can vary from one office to another.

This section will be a convenient reference for the new assistant or for the assistant who has not worked in the field for some time.

BANDAGING

1. Assemble all supplies before entering the patient's room.

2. Prepare the skin for bandaging. Clean wound site and surrounding area and make sure area is completely dry.

3. Always place a sterile dressing over an open wound before applying the wrap.

4. Always anchor the bandage. (This will help keep it from slipping.)

5. Keep body part surfaces from touching each other if possible. (Put a piece of gauze in between the surfaces. This will help keep the skin from becoming irritated.)

6. The body part that is to be bandaged should be placed in its normal position.

7. Bandages should always be applied in a distal to proximal motion.

8. At the end of the procedure, check with the patient to see how the bandage feels. It should not be so tight that it cuts off circulation, but it should not be so loose that it falls off.

The patient should be given an information form about how to take care of his or her wound. Other information on the form should include what symptoms the patient should be alerted to, medication directions, and the date of the follow-up appointment.

BANDAGING EXAMPLES

How to Anchor a Bandage

Recurrent Turn on a Finger

How to Apply a Sling

(continued on following page)

9

BANDAGING *(continued from previous page)*

Tube Gauze Bandage

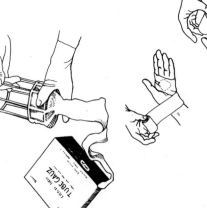

Closed Spiral Bandage

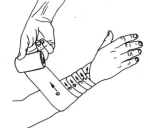

Open Spiral Bandage

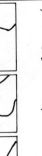

Figure Eight Turn

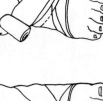

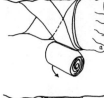

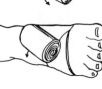

Any Modifications: _____

Physician's Approval: _____

EAR IRRIGATION/LAVAGE

ITEMS NECESSARY

1. Mineral oil (Sometimes necessary to soften cerumen prior to procedure; leave in 10-15 minutes before attempting to irrigate.)
2. Irrigating solution (i.e., peroxide, water, etc.)
3. Basin for solution
4. Irrigator (May use a metal syringe or a rubber bulb syringe.)
5. 6" Cotton-tipped applicators
6. Otoscope and ear speculum
7. Towel
8. Ear basin
9. Tissues
10. Latex gloves
11. Cotton balls/gauze pads

Other supplies:

FACTS AND TROUBLESHOOTING TIPS

1. View the ear with an otoscope to determine the location of the obstruction before attempting to irrigate.
2. If the patient appears to have a lot of cerumen, try inserting peroxide or mineral oil to help soften the cerumen before the procedure begins. (Check with the physician first.)
3. Place a waterproof barrier over the patient's shoulder to keep the patient from getting wet.
4. Irrigating solution should be warmed to body temperature before irrigation takes place.
5. After filling the syringe, always expel air from it before attempting to irrigate. This will help decrease the risk of possible eardrum damage.
6. For an adult, gently pull the auricle up and back. For a child, pull back, and for a young child or infant, pull down and back.
7. To avoid severe pain and damage to the eardrum, direct the flow of the solution toward the sides of the ear canal instead of forcing it directly into the middle of the ear.
8. If the patient appears to be in discomfort while doing the procedure, stop and alert the physician before attempting to go any further.

Any Modifications:

Physician's Approval:

9

ELECTROCARDIOGRAMS

EQUIPMENT

EKG machine	EKG paper	Electrodes	Electrolyte	Mounting paper

LEAD PLACEMENT FOR A STANDARD 12 LEAD EKG

Limb Placement

Fleshy portion of right upper arm	Fleshy portion of left upper arm	Inner portion of right lower leg	Inner portion of left lower leg

Chest Placement

V-1 4th intercostal space right of sternum	V-2 4th intercostal space left of sternum	V-3 Midpoint between V-2 and V-4	V-4 5th intercostal space midclavicular	V-5 Anterior axillary, on the same plane as V-4	V-6 Mid-axillary, on the same plane as V-4 and V-5

STANDARD LEAD MARKINGS

Lead I	Lead II	Lead III	AVR	AVL	AVF
•	• •	• • •	–	– –	– – –

V-1	V-2	V-3	V-4	V-5	V-6
– •	– • •	– • • •	– • • • •	– • • • • •	– • • • • • •

ARTIFACT ILLUSTRATIONS

Wandering Baseline	Somatic Interference	Alternating Current	Interrupted Baseline

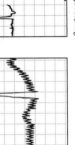

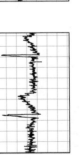

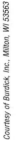

Courtesy of Burdick, Inc., Milton, WI 53563

EKG Tips

1. Explain the procedure in detail to the patient. This will help relieve any anxiety the patient might be feeling.
2. Dimming the light in the room might help the patient relax more.
3. Try to choose a table that will fit the patient.
4. If the patient is missing a limb, place the electrode on the stump above any scarring.

CAUSES OF EKG ARTIFACTS

Wandering Baseline	Somatic Interference	Alternating Current	Interrupted Baseline
Electrodes that are dirty or corroded	Uncomfortable patient	Lead wires do not follow the body contour	A broken lead wire
Electrolyte distribution is unequal	A physical condition, such as Parkinson's disease	The EKG unit is not grounded or improperly grounded	The patient cable is broken
The patient has body lotion or oil on his or her skin	Movement of the patient	Corroded or dirty electrodes	
The electrodes are put on too tightly or too loosely	The patient is nervous	The presence of other electrical equipment in the room (i.e., fluorescent lighting)	

FACTS AND TROUBLESHOOTING TIPS

Paper Sensitivity	Abnormal Beats or Rhythm	Paper Speed
The sensitivity is normally run at I mv/10 mm	If any abnormal beats are noted while running an EKG, check with the physician to see if he or she wants to run a rhythm strip at the end of the reading.	Normal paper speed is set at 25 mm/sec
The sensitivity should be turned down to 1/2 when the R wave is going off the graph. (Try to adjust the position control knob either up or down before changing the sensitivity.)	If an abnormal rhythm is noted while running an EKG, check with the physician to see if he or she wants to run a rhythm strip at the end of the reading.	If the patient has an abnormally fast heart rate, turn the paper speed up to 50 mm/sec to give a more defined complex.
The sensitivity should be on double standard when the beats are barely visible. Be sure to standardize whenever the position control knob is turned.		

A good standardization should be 10 mm high and 2 mm wide.

Always read the manufacturer's instructions before doing an EKG. No two models are the same, and it is important to understand how to run the unit before attempting to complete the EKG.

(continued on following page)

ELECTROCARDIOGRAMS *(continued from previous page)*

Any Modifications:

_____

_____

_____

_____

Physician's Approval: _____

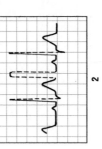

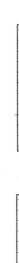

1

SENSITIVITY CONTROL

1/2

2

Courtesy of Burdick, Inc., Milton, WI 53563

EYE IRRIGATION/LAVAGE

ITEMS NECESSARY

1. Irrigating solution ordered by doctor (sterile)
2. 10 cc bulb syringe (sterile)
3. Towels
4. Eye basin
5. Tissues
6. Sterile basin to hold solution
7. Latex gloves
8. Waterproof drape

Other supplies:

_____

_____

_____

FACTS AND TROUBLESHOOTING TIPS

1. Set up supplies and equipment in order of use.

2. Warm the irrigating solution to body temperature (98.6° F).

3. Inspect each eye to determine the location of the foreign body or the condition of the eye.

4. Drape a waterproof barrier over the front part of the body to help keep the patient from getting wet.

5. Use a gauze square to pull down the lower lid. This will help keep fingers from slipping.

6. Try to position the patient so the solution will not run into the unaffected eye. The affected eye should be positioned downward. (This will help prevent cross-infection.)

7. Always irrigate from the inner canthus of the eye to the outer canthus.

8. Do not allow the syringe to touch the eye. This will help avoid infection and injury.

9. Wipe excess solution from eye and carefully reexamine it to ensure that the irrigation has produced the desired result.

10. Record the irrigation and results on the patient's chart.

Any Modifications: _____

_____

_____

_____

_____

_____

Physician's Approval: _____

9

INTRADERMAL INJECTION

SUPPLIES

Medication   Needle   Syringe   Alcohol   Cotton   Gloves   Adhesive Bandage   Sharp's container

NEEDLE AND SYRINGE SIZE

Syringe: Tuberculin (1 cc)   Needle gauge: 26-27 G   Needle length: 3/8-1/2"

INJECTION SITES

Anterior forearm   Mid-back

MEDICATIONS ROUTINELY GIVEN BY THIS ROUTE

Allergy skin tests   TB skin testing medication

ANGLE USED

10-15 degree angle

ULTIMATE GOAL OF INJECTION

To form a wheal

FACTS AND TROUBLESHOOTING TIPS

1. The amount of medication administered by this route is usually between 0.01-0.2 ccs.

2. Stretching the skin will permit the medication to be injected more easily.

3. Allow alcohol to dry before injecting the medication. (This will prevent the tissue from becoming irritated by the alcohol.).

4. If bevel is not in an upward position, a wheal will not be able to form.

5. Be careful to go just under the skin and no further to ensure that the dermal layer of the skin is being entered.

6. Do not massage the area or apply an adhesive bandage following the injection. This could result in dispersing the medication into the deeper layers of tissue.

7. Once the injection is given, many physicians will have the assistant draw a circle around the wheal, for later comparative studies.

8. Notify the physician immediately if patient has an anaphylactic reaction during or following the injection.

   Have epinephrine or equivalent standing by. (Never administer any medication without a direct order from the physician.)

9. Allergy Testing: Patient should always wait for results. TB Skin Testing: Patient will need to have testing site read in a 48-72-hour time frame, depending on the method that is used.

Any Modifications: _____

_____

Physician's Approval:_____

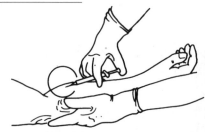

INTRAMUSCULAR INJECTION (DELTOID)

SUPPLIES

Medication   Needle   Syringe   Alcohol   Cotton   Gloves   Adhesive bandage   Sharp's container

NEEDLE AND SYRINGE SIZE

Syringe size (1-2 cc, depending on the amount of medication being administered); Needle sizes: small frame, adult/very little adipose tissue (25 G 5/8" needle); average frame, adult/average amount of adipose tissue (22-23 G, 1" needle); large frame, considerable amount of adipose tissue (22-23 G, 1 1/2"-2" needle), depending on the amount of fat. *The deltoid should never be considered in an infant or small child.* (Needle sizes will vary from office to office. Check with the physician to see what he or she prefers.)

ANGLE

90 degrees

INJECTION LOCATION

The deltoid can be found by placing the finger on the tip of the acromion process and measuring three fingers down. The outline of the deltoid can be viewed in most patients by having them extend their arm outward and away from the body. The injection should be administered in the center of the deltoid whenever possible.

MEDICATIONS ROUTINELY GIVEN BY THIS ROUTE

IM injections, which are water-based or thin in viscosity and measure less than 2 ccs, i.e., adult immunizations.

FACTS AND TROUBLESHOOTING TIPS

1. Never attempt to give any medication that is more than 2 ccs, oil-based, or thick in viscosity, using this muscle. The deltoid is a small muscle and will not be able to absorb it. (Check the medication's package insert to be certain.)

2. Always make sure the alcohol is dry before inserting the needle. (The alcohol can irritate the tissue and cause discomfort to the patient.)

3. Be sure to hold the skin tautly when inserting the needle to ensure that the needle gets into the muscle.

4. Never dart the injection. (This will traumatize the tissue and cause more pain to the patient.)

5. If blood enters the syringe upon aspiration, withdraw the needle and start over.

6. A tight sleeve can constrict the arm and cause excessive bleeding from the puncture site.

7. Inject the medication steadily and slowly. Pushing the medication in too fast can destroy tissue and cause discomfort to the patient.

8. Withdraw the needle quickly and at the same angle it entered. This will help reduce the patient's discomfort.

9. Be sure to gently massage the injection site. Massaging too vigorously will cause the patient discomfort and possible irritation to the tissues.

10. Report any unusual symptoms.

11. When given antibiotics, the patient should wait a minimum of 20 minutes before leaving the facility because of the possibility of an anaphylactic reaction. Have epinephrine or an equivalent standing by, just in case. Never give any medication without a direct order from the physician!

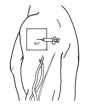

Any Modifications:

Physician's Approval:

INTRAMUSCULAR INJECTION (DORSOGLUTEAL)

SUPPLIES

Medication   Needle   Syringe   Alcohol   Cotton   Gloves   Adhesive bandage   Sharp's container

NEEDLE AND SYRINGE SIZE

The gauge will depend on how thick the medication is. Thicker medications will usually take a larger gauge, such as 18-20 G. Thinner medications can take a smaller gauge, such as 21-22 G. Needle lengths will vary according to the size of the patient. Smaller framed adults/very little adipose tissue (1" needle); average framed adults/average amount of adipose tissue (1 1/2" needle); larger framed adults/moderate amount of adipose tissue (2-3" needle). Syringe size will vary according to the amount of medication being injected, usually a 3-5 cc syringe. This site is not recommended for infants or small children. The vastus lateralis is a much safer site for this age group. (Needle sizes will vary from office to office; check with the physician to see what he or she prefers.)

ANGLE

90 degrees

MEDICATIONS ROUTINELY GIVEN BY THIS ROUTE

Medications that are greater than 2 ccs, oil-based, or thick in viscosity. Examples include steroid and hormone injections and antibiotics like penicillin. (Check package insert to be certain.)

INJECTION LOCATION

The injection is given in the upper outer quadrant of the gluteal area. For the exact location, draw an imaginary line from the greater trochanter to the posterior superior iliac spine and go above and to the outside of that area.

FACTS AND TROUBLESHOOTING TIPS

1. Be very careful to stay in the area that was described under Injection Location. Straying from that area could result in hitting the sciatic nerve, which could cause an extensive amount of pain or even paralysis. BE CAREFUL!

2. The patient should lie on his or her abdomen with toes pointed inward, or should bend over and take the weight off the side where he or she is receiving the injection. (This aids in the relaxation of the gluteal muscles.)

3. Always make sure the alcohol is dry before inserting the needle. (The alcohol can irritate the tissue and cause discomfort to the patient.)

4. If blood enters the syringe upon aspiration, withdraw the needle and start over.

5. Inject the medication slowly and steadily. Pushing the medication in too quickly can destroy tissue and cause discomfort to the patient.

6. Withdraw the needle quickly and at the same angle it entered to help reduce patient discomfort.

7. Gently massage the injection site. Be careful not to massage too vigorously as this could irritate the tissues further.

8. When administering antibiotics, the patient should wait a minimum of 20 minutes before leaving the facility, due to a possible anaphylactic reaction. Have epinephrine or an equivalent standing by, just in case. Never give any medication without a direct order from the physician!

9. Be sure to report any unusual symptoms.

Any Modifications:

_____

_____

_____

_____

_____

Physician's Approval:_____

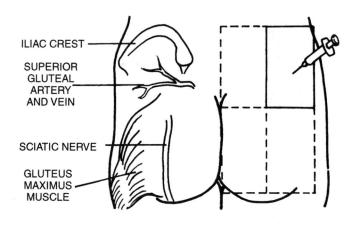

ILIAC CREST

SUPERIOR
GLUTEAL
ARTERY
AND VEIN

SCIATIC NERVE

GLUTEUS
MAXIMUS
MUSCLE

INTRAMUSCULAR PEDIATRIC INJECTION

COMMON SITES

Vastus Lateralis	Dorsogluteal	Deltoid
1. Located on the front surface of the mid-thigh, away from major blood vessels and nerves.	Draw an imaginary line between the greater trochanter and the posterior superior iliac spine. Stay above and to the outside of this area.	This site can be found by placing a finger on the tip of the acromion process and measuring down approximately three fingers.
2. This site is recommended from birth through young childhood.	This muscle should not be used until the child is walking.	Not recommended in infants and small children because the muscle is too small to absorb very much medication. Using this site may cause more pain for the patient.
3. The size of the thigh will dictate the length of the needle.	Movement and squirming of the child may cause the assistant to accidentally hit the sciatic nerve. This could result in excruciating pain to the patient as well as possible paralysis.	The muscle mass should be grasped at the site where the needle is going to enter the the skin and compressed between the thumb and fingers.
4. The skin should be compressed between thumb and fingers. Be sure that the leg is secured so that the child cannot move.	In cases where the child cannot be secured, it is best to ask for assistance from a coworker or parent.	Angle 90°, but needle should be tilted upward slightly toward the top of the arm or shoulder.
5. Angle 90°	Angle 90°	

IMPORTANT TIPS

1. The length of the needle will depend on the size of the muscle to be used.
2. The gauge of the needle will depend on the viscosity of the medication.
3. Never tell children that the injection is not going to hurt; instead, tell them they may feel a little sting.
4. Reward children after the injection is completed.

(continued on next page)

INTRAMUSCULAR PEDIATRIC INJECTION *(continued from previous page)*

5. Be sure to accurately chart medication on the progress note. There is usually a place on the cover of the chart to record the injection as well. In many cases it will be necessary to document immunizations in an immunization log.

6. Never give medication without a direct order from the physician.

7. Always have the parent sign the immunization authorization form *before* the injection is given.

8. Always verify medication allergies!

Any Modifications:

_____

_____

_____

_____

Physician's Approval: _____

SUBCUTANEOUS INJECTION

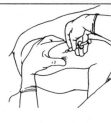

SUPPLIES

Medication	Needle	Syringe	Alcohol	Cotton	Gloves	Adhesive bandage	Sharp's container

NEEDLE AND SYRINGE SIZE

Syringe: Insulin, Tuberculin or 2-3 cc syringe   Needle Gauge: 25-27 G   Needle Length: 3/8-5/8"

INJECTION SITES

Upper arm (under the deltoid, circulating around to the back of the arm)   Thigh   Back   Abdomen (Any portion of the body where there is fat.)

MEDICATION EXAMPLES ROUTINELY GIVEN BY THIS ROUTE

Insulin, Allergy Injections, MMR Immunization, Epinephrine

ANGLE USED

45-90 degrees (ask physician what his or her specifications are)

FACTS AND TROUBLESHOOTING TIPS

1. Elderly and dehydrated patients will have less subcutaneous tissue, thus it is important to use a smaller-sized needle on those types of patients.

2. Medications that exceed more than 2 ccs, are viscid, or irritating to the tissue, should not be given by this route.

3. Avoid using sites that are grossly adipose, inflamed, hardened, or swollen.

4. Allow the area to completely dry after applying the alcohol. (Alcohol can irritate the tissue.)

5. Do not inject the medication too quickly. (This could destroy the tissue and cause the patient discomfort.)

6. Gently massage the area after medication is inserted. (Vigorous massaging will cause irritation to the tissue.)

7. Make sure the patient waits a minimum of twenty minutes following an allergy shot. (The patient could have an anaphylactic reaction.) Have epinephrine or an equivalent standing by. Never administer any medication without a direct order from the physician!

8. Check the patient before he or she leaves. Record any problems that might have developed following the injection, i.e., wheal, erythema, edema, unusual pain, etc.

Any Modifications: _____

Physician's Approval: _____

POSITIONING

The following diagrams illustrate the various positions that are used for different exams and describe the instances where a patient may be placed in those positions.

POSITIONS

Name and Type	Description	Special Instructions	Illustration
Dorsal Recumbent Abdominal exams Vaginal exams Rectal exams	Patient is placed in a supine position with back flat on the table, legs flexed.	Try to make the patient comfortable by placing a pillow under the head. A sheet may be draped over the patient to provide warmth and modesty. (Use a diamond-shaped drape for a vaginal or rectal exam.)	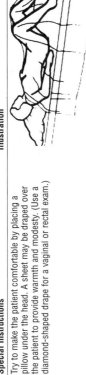
Horizontal Recumbent Anterior surface exams Various Xrays	Patient lies in a supine position or flat on back (if possible).	Same as dorsal recumbent	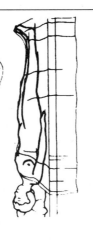
Dorsal Lithotomy Vaginal exams Rectal exams	Patient is placed in a supine position, feet are placed in stirrups, and legs are spread apart.	Place pillow under the patient's head. Place a diamond-shaped drape over the patient. Make sure the patient's buttocks are even with the bottom edge of the table.	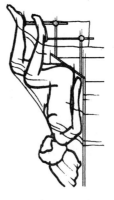

(continued on following page)

9

POSITIONING *(continued from previous page)*

Name and Type	Description	Special Instructions	Illustration
Prone Position Back or spine exams	Patient lies flat on stomach with arms folded out to the sides.	Patient may need pillow for comfort. Place drape over patient to provide warmth and modesty.	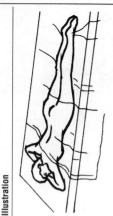
Sims or Left Lateral Certain Xrays Rectal exam Enema Sigmoidoscopies	Patient is placed on left side with right knee flexed upward toward the chest.	Patient may need pillow for comfort. Place drape over patient to provide warmth and modesty. (Use diamond-shaped drape for rectal exam.)	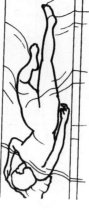
Knee-Chest Rectal exams Sigmoidoscopies	Patient should be placed in a kneeling position, knees should be drawn toward chest and spread slightly apart. Arms are flexed and placed under head.	This is a very difficult position to maintain. Give patient clear instructions. Place a pillow underneath the patient's head. Use a diamond-shaped drape.	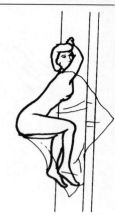

(continued on following page)

POSITIONING *(continued from previous page)*

Name and Type	Description	Special Instructions	Illustration
Fowler's Position Respiratory discomfort Cardiovascular problems Back problems	Patient sits perfectly upright at a 90-degree angle.	Make sure the patient is secure. Many tables will have a belt to lock the patient in. Provide a drape for warmth and modesty.	
Semi-Fowler's Same as Fowler's	Same as Fowler's only patient's back is at a 45-degree angle.	Same as Fowler's	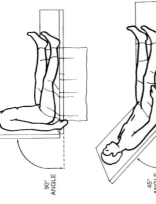
Trendelenberg Shock Fainting	Patient is in a supine position with feet elevated. (Use pillows if table cannot be placed in this position.)	Be sure patient is secure and locked in. Monitor patient carefully. Alert physician to any complications. A full drape may be used.	

Physician's Approval: _____

SURGICAL PROCEDURES

Items Directly on the Field	Items Off to the Side of the Field	Facts/Tips
Needle/syringe	Bandaging materials/antiseptic cream	Arrange items in order of use.
Cotton-tip applicators	Bandage scissors	Check expiration dates of sterile items/medications.
Disposable fenestrated towels	Adhesive tape	Remind patient to empty bladder prior to procedure.
Gauze squares	Sterile irrigation solution	Prepare set-up just before the physician comes in to prevent possible contamination.
Appropriate suture	Antiseptic swabs/solution	Adjust lighting according to the location of the injury.
Towel clamps	Alcohol/cotton balls	Have any prescriptions ready the physician may want to prescribe to the patient. i.e., antibiotic/analgesic.
Scalpel handle/blade	Latex gloves (physician/assistant) Keep plenty of gloves handy	Make sure the patient read, understood, and signed the surgery consent form prior to the procedure.
Tissue forceps	Biohazard sharps (container/bag)	Check on patient continuously throughout the procedure.
Needle driver/holder	Biopsy request form/biopsy container	Assistant will usually bandage the area involved, following the surgery.
Hemostats	Patient's chart	Give the patient written instructions regarding home care.
Surgical scissors	Mayo stand/sterile drape	Help the patient to the reception area.
Retractor	Anesthetic	Have the patient schedule a follow-up appointment.
Thumb forceps	PPE (Face shield/mask/gown)	
Sterile solution holders (2)	Hyfrecator/cautery unit, (physician's preference)	

Any Modifications:

Physician's Approval:

BLOOD PRESSURE

EQUIPMENT

Sphygmomanometer · Stethoscope · Alcohol wipes

Blood pressure measures the amount of force exerted by the blood on the arterial walls. Systolic pressure measures the pressure of the blood against the arterial walls as the heart contracts. This represents the highest point of blood pressure. Diastolic pressure measures the pressure of the blood against the arterial walls when the heart is relaxing. This represents the lowest pressure point.

KOROTKOFF SOUNDS

Phase I	Phase II	Phase III	Phase IV	Phase V
When first faint but clear beat is heard.	The sound appears to be swishy.	When sounds increase in intensity (crisper).	When sound becomes muffled.	The point at which the sound disappears.

NORMAL BLOOD PRESSURE RANGE FOR VARIOUS AGE GROUPS

AVERAGE BLOOD PRESSURE RANGE

AGE RANGE	
Adult	120/80 (or a range of 90-140 systolic, and 60-90 diastolic)
14-17 years of age	120/76
8-13 years of age	110/72
2-7 years of age	100/64
1 year	94/64

FACTORS THAT AFFECT BLOOD PRESSURE

Exercise	Age	Gender	Body Position	Medications
Physical activity or exercise will temporarily increase blood pressure. (Allow the patient to rest before taking his or her blood pressure.)	As age increases, blood pressure also increases.	Adult males usually have a higher blood pressure than adult females.	Blood pressure will vary according to what position the patient is in. Document position if other than sitting. L (lying), St (standing).	Many medications will alter blood pressure. (List all medications being taken by the patient.)

The time of day blood pressure is taken will have a significant effect. The lowest reading is normally in the morning because of decreased metabolism. Other factors that alter blood pressure include emotional states, pain, if the patient recently ate, bladder distention, smoking, medications (OTC and prescribed), street drugs, and alcohol.

(continued on following page)

BLOOD PRESSURE *(continued from previous page)*

FACTS AND TROUBLESHOOTING TIPS

1. Use the appropriate size cuff for the patient's body frame.

2. Make sure that mercury is on zero for mercury cuffs and that the dial is on zero for aneroid cuffs before pumping up the cuff.

3. Deflate the cuff approximately 2-3 mmHg/second.

4. Beware of auscultary gap (silent interval between systolic and diastolic pressure). This can be avoided by using the palpatory method of taking blood pressure before attempting the auscultary method.

Palpatory Method:

1. Palpate brachial or radial arteries in each arm. (Select the arm with the stronger pulse.)

2. Wrap cuff smoothly, "snugly," around arm with the center of the cuff over the brachial artery.

3. Determine the maximum inflation by palpating the radial pulse and inflating the cuff until the pulse is no longer felt.

4. Deflate cuff.

5. Mentally add 30 mm to the reading. That number is what the cuff will be pumped up to when the blood pressure is taken.

5. Do not take blood pressure through clothes.

6. Make sure arm is at heart level when taking blood pressure.

7. Wait a minimum of 15 seconds before reattempting to take blood pressure in the same arm (maximum of 3 times).

8. Record in which arm the blood pressure was taken, as well as what position the patient was in, if other than a sitting position.

9. Provide support for the patient's arm(s) during the procedure.

Any Modifications: _____

_____

_____

_____

Physician's Approval: _____

PULSE

Radial Pulse	Apical Pulse	Brachial Pulse	Carotid Pulse	Pedal Pulse
Located on the inner portion of the wrist, just below the thumb.	Located at the 5th intercostal space, just to the left of the midclavicular line (apex location).	Located in the antecubital space.	Located on the front side of the neck, just slightly to one side or the other.	Located on the upper surface of the foot, midpoint between the 1st and 2nd metatarsal bones.
Use index and great finger to measure the radial pulse.	Use a stethoscope to measure an apical pulse (listen to the beats).	Use index and middle fingers to measure the brachial pulse.	Use index and middle fingers to measure the carotid pulse.	Use index and middle fingers to measure a pedal pulse.
Most commonly used method.	Used when the pulse is hard to palpate and routinely used on infants and children < 3 years old.	Used when taking blood pressures and on infants in CPR situations.	Used in CPR situations and routinely used by athletes after a workout.	Used to assess circulation of the foot.

PULSE RATES

Age Range	Average Pulse
Age 13-Adulthood	80
Age 6-12	95
Age 2-6	100
Age 1-2	105
1 Month – 12 Months	110
Newborn to 1 Month	140

	Pulse Range
	60-100
	75-110
	75-120
	80-130
	80-140
	120-160

FACTORS THAT AFFECT PULSE

Age	Gender	Medications	Exercise	Metabolism
As age increases, pulse rate decreases.	Females have a faster pulse rate than do males.	Medications will cause the pulse rate to be altered. Stimulants increase the pulse rate, whereas depressants decrease the pulse rate.	Physical activity will cause the pulse rate to rise.	An increase in body metabolism, i.e., fever and pregnancy.

EMOTIONS CAN ALSO AFFECT PULSE RATE!

(continued on following page)

PULSE *(continued from previous page)*

APICAL-RADIAL PULSE

1. One person obtains the radial pulse at the same time another person is obtaining an apical pulse.

2. Subtract the radial pulse rate from the apical pulse rate. This is determined as the pulse deficit.

FACTS AND TROUBLESHOOTING TIPS

Record if pulse is normal, full or bounding, weak or thready. Record any arrhythmias. Keep fingers on pulse site while measuring respiration, so the patient will not be aware that you are measuring his or her respiration rate. (This will help keep the patient from altering his or her respiration rate.)

Any Modifications: _____

_____

_____

_____

_____

_____

Physician's Approval: _____

RESPIRATION

Various Breath Sounds

Wheezing	Crackles (Rales)	Stertor	Stridor	Gurgles
Continuous high-pitched sounds. (Patient really struggles for breath.)	Intermittent sounds that can be wet or dry and vary in pitch. (Need stethoscope.)	Sounds like the patient is snoring upon respiration.	High-pitched crowing sound, heard during inspiration. (Common in croup.)	Constant low-pitched wheezing, especially during exhalation. (Need stethoscope.)

RESPIRATION NORMALS

Age Range	Normal Range	Age Range	Normal Range
Infant	30-50/minute	16-18 years	16-20/minute
1-2 years	20-40/minute	Adulthood	16-20/minute
10-16 years	17-22/minute		

FACTORS THAT AFFECT RESPIRATION RATE

Age	Illness	Drugs	Exercise	Emotions
As age increases, respiration decreases.	Fever causes respiration rate to rise.	Drugs can alter respiration rate.	Exercise increases respiration rate.	Emotions can alter respiration rate. (Usually they increase it.)

RHYTHM AND DEPTH

RHYTHM

1. Respiration rhythms should be regular and equal.
2. The pauses between inspiration and expiration also should be equal.
3. Any variation in rhythm should be listed.

DEPTH

1. Depth should not vary from one respiration to the next.
2. Record depth as shallow, normal, or deep.

COMMON TERMINOLOGY

Hyperpnea	Hypopnea	Tachypnea	Bradypnea	Apnea
Deep and rapid respirations (Panting)	Very shallow (1/2 normal volume)	Rapid respirations	Slow respirations	Temporary absence of respirations

(continued on following page)

RESPIRATION *(continued from previous page)*

COMMON TERMINOLOGY

Orthopnea	Cyanosis	Eupnea
Can breathe easier in a sitting or standing position.	Bluish discoloration of the skin, lips, and nail beds.	Normal breathing

FACTS AND TROUBLESHOOTING TIPS

1. Take respiration without the patient's knowledge, best done immediately following taking the pulse, while fingers are still palpating radial artery.
2. One complete inhalation and one complete exhalation equals one respiration.
3. If respiration is irregular, take for one full minute, otherwise you may check for 30 seconds and multiply by 2.

Any Modifications: _____

_____

_____

_____

_____

Physician's Approval: _____

TEMPERATURE

	Location	Average Range	Glass Thermometer (Timing)	Facts
Oral:	Should be placed under the tongue and off to the side of the frenulum linguae.	97.6° F-99.6° F (37° C)	3–7 minutes	Most common method used. Instruct patient to keep mouth closed at all times. Should not use this method on young or mentally impaired patients because of safety issues.
Axillary:	Place directly under the armpit, centered in the middle.	96.6° F-98.6° F (37.6° C)	5–10 minutes	Least accurate method used. Most common method for infants and young children. Keep arm closed against body.
Rectal:	Infants: Insert thermometer about 1/2" into anal canal. Children: Insert thermometer about 1" into anal canal. Adults: Insert thermometer about 1 1/2" into anal canal.	98.6° F-100.6° F (36.4° C)	3–5 minutes	Use lubrication for most types of thermometers. Follow manufacturer's instructions when using digital or chemical thermometers. The anus can be found easily in the infant by placing infant on its back with its ankles in the air. Adult patients should be put in supine position. Never force thermometer into the anal canal!

TEMPERATURE RANGES VARY FROM REFERENCE TO REFERENCE, SO THE LOWEST–HIGHEST TEMPERATURE RANGES ARE PROVIDED. (Check with physician!)

	Location	Average Range	Glass Thermometer (Timing)	Facts
Aural:	Place covered probe into ear canal, sealing the opening.	97.6° F-99.6° F (37° C)	Within seconds	Saves time! (Follow manufacturer's instructions.)

FACTORS THAT INFLUENCE TEMPERATURE

Time of Day	Age	Patient's Normal Temperature	Environment	Pregnancy
Lowest in the morning.	The younger the patient, the lower the body temperature.	Always review the chart to see what temperature the patient normally runs.	The cooler the room, the lower the body temperature.	Usually higher during pregnancy, because of increased metabolism.

STRONG EMOTIONS WILL ALSO CAUSE BODY TEMPERATURE TO ELEVATE.

(continued on following page)

TEMPERATURE *(continued from previous page)*

TYPES OF FEVER

REMITTENT FEVER	INTERMITTENT FEVER	CONTINUOUS FEVER
A wide range of temperature fluctuations, usually above normal. Typically seen during attacks of influenza, endocarditis, and pneumonia.	The temperature rises and falls, often going from high to normal and even subnormal at times. Typically seen during viral and bacterial infections.	The temperature stays elevated over an extended period with little fluctuation. Typically seen during scarlet fever episodes and certain types of pneumonia.

FACTS AND TROUBLESHOOTING TIPS

1. Always shake thermometer below 96° F when using mercury thermometer.
2. Record reading in even numbers when using mercury thermometer.
3. Always check expiration date of disposable thermometers.
4. Use a new sheath for each patient.
5. Follow manufacturer's instructions when using automated or chemical thermometers.
6. Wait a minimum of 15-30 minutes after the patient has eaten, drank, chewed gum, or smoked before doing a temperature, or false results will be produced.

Equipment: Thermometer, Sheaths, (Rectal temperature, add lubricant and gloves)

TEMPERATURE CONVERSIONS

To convert **Celsius to Fahrenheit:**

1. C × 9/5 + 32

Example: 37° C × 9/5 = (333/5) or 66.6 + 32 = 98.6° F

To convert **Fahrenheit to Celsius:**

1. F−32 x 5/9

Example: 98.6° F − 32 = 66.6 × 5/9 = (333/9) or 37° C

Any Modifications: _____

_____

Physician's Approval: _____

CAPILLARY SPECIMEN COLLECTION FACTS

SUPPLIES

Disposable gloves   Alcohol or antiseptic wipes   Cotton balls or gauze pads   Sterile lancet or automatic lancet   Biohazard container

WHEN METHOD IS USED

1. When only a small portion of blood is necessary.
2. When collecting most infant specimens.
3. When doing PKUs.
4. When a hematocrit and/or hemoglobin only is ordered.
5. When doing blood glucose level with a glucose meter.

FACTS AND TROUBLESHOOTING TIPS

1. Warming the site before the procedure will help dilate the blood vessels so the patient will bleed more easily. (Disregard this practice if the patient is on anticoagulation therapy.)
2. The use of an automatic lancet is encouraged in most cases, because the depth of penetration can be controlled better and there is usually less pain associated with the stick.
3. The use of a regular lancet is encouraged when the skin is very thick or calloused.
4. When doing a finger stick, the middle and ring finger are better choices, because the index finger and thumb are usually more calloused.
5. When puncturing the finger, the assistant should stick the lateral portion of the tip, as this is the least sensitive part of the finger.
6. The puncture should go against the grain of the finger, or to a right angle of the lines that form the fingerprints.
7. The puncture should be at least 2-3 mm deep.
8. Allow alcohol to completely dry before puncturing finger. This will help prevent hemolysis. (Wet alcohol can cause hemolysis.)
9. Always remember to wipe away the first drop of blood. (This will help ensure a more accurate specimen.)
10. If the site stops bleeding, try reapplying alcohol to the area. Wipe away the first drop of blood and reapply gentle pressure.
11. Squeezing the finger while collecting a capillary sample can lead to inaccurate test results. (This is so because tissue fluid can mix with the specimen and produce a false reading.)

(continued on following page)

CAPILLARY SPECIMEN COLLECTION FACTS *(continued from previous page)*

COMMON SITES

Great or Ring Finger	The Heel of an Infant	The Earlobe

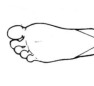

Any Modifications: _____

_____

_____

Physician's Approval: _____

HEMATOCRIT

SUPPLIES

Protective equipment	Centrifuge	Biohazard container	Gloves	Sterile lancet	Alcohol	Cotton balls	Sealing compound	Capillary tubes

SITES WHERE BLOOD FOR HEMATOCRIT MAY BE OBTAINED

The great or ring finger, or heel of infant

PURPOSE OF TEST

Measures the packed red blood cell volume, and checks for anemia

FACTS AND TROUBLESHOOTING TIPS

1. Be sure to wipe away the first drop of blood before starting to fill capillary tubes.

2. Calibrated tubes should be filled to the calibration line.

3. Avoid getting air bubbles into the tube.

4. Do not allow the tube to rest against a finger. This will close off the opening of the pipette and will not allow the blood to enter it.

5. Always fill two tubes.

6. Be sure to completely seal one end only of the capillary tube with sealing compound.

7. Always balance centrifuge by placing tubes directly across from each other.

8. Be sure to place the tubes so the sealed end is toward the the outside of the centrifuge, or blood will run out of the tubes and into the centrifuge.

9. Be sure to lock the cover tightly onto the centrifuge before spinning. (If this is not done, the tubes may break.)

10. Check the manufacturer's instructions to learn how to operate the unit. (Most hematocrits are run at 10,000 rpm for 3-5 minutes.)

11. If results vary more than two numbers between the two tubes, the test should be repeated. (This will not always be possible.)

12. In most cases, the hematocrit should match the hemoglobin once the hemoglobin is multiplied by 3. (This should be within a + or − 3 deviation.)

(continued on following page)

HEMATOCRIT *(continued from previous page)*

HOW TO READ A HEMATOCRIT

1. Line the top of the plasma over the 100% mark.

2. The bottom of the cell column (just above the sealing compound) should be placed on the zero line.

3. The results should be read where the scale corresponds to the top of the packed red cell volume.

Any Modifications:

_____

_____

_____

_____

_____

Physician's Approval: _____

PLASMA

BUFFY COAT

READ THIS LINE AT THE MENISCUS FOR HCT%

SHOULD BE LINED UP IN CENTRIFUGE AT "0" (ZERO)

CLAY SEALANT

PHLEBOTOMY TIPS

1. If the patient has had a history of fainting during phlebotomy procedures or appears apprehensive, it is wise to have the patient lie down during the procedure.

2. Always ask the patient from which arm they prefer to have blood drawn. (The assistant should observe and feel the patient's arm to palpate the vein to determine the best site.) Nine times out of ten the patient knows best.

3. The median cephalic vein is usually the vein of choice. This can be found in the center of the antecubital space in both arms.

4. When no veins are visible or palpable in the arms, go to the hands.

5. Do not attempt to enter veins that are scarred, burned, bruised, or close to areas where infection is present. If patient already complains of soreness or pain in a particular area, avoid that area as well.

6. If the vein starts to swell while the needle is being inserted into the patient's arm, remove the tourniquet and withdraw the needle immediately.

7. Remove the tourniquet before the needle to minimize internal and external bleeding at the puncture site. (Release tourniquet on first or second tube if possible.)

8. Pop the tube before withdrawing the needle. This will help avoid blood dripping onto the patient.

9. Do not delay in transferring the blood from the syringe into the tubes, or clotting may occur.

10. Apply gentle pressure for a minimum of two to three minutes following a blood draw, and elevate the arm to minimize the risks of bruising or acquiring a hematoma. (If the patient is on anticoagulant therapy, apply pressure for a minimum of five minutes or more.)

11. Never stick a patient more than twice. Some offices have a one-time rule. Check with the supervising physician to learn about office procedure.

12. Use a blood pressure cuff instead of a tourniquet, and use a needle that is 1 1/2" long on patients who are obese.

13. If the patient's veins collapse easily, use the smallest blood tube (7 ml or less) that is allowed by the lab. You may consider using a syringe or butterfly.

14. Never leave the tourniquet on for more than two minutes.

15. Dispose of needles in a Sharp's container.

16. Any articles that are saturated with blood should be disposed of in a biohazard container.

HEMOLYSIS PREVENTION TIPS

1. Vacuum tubes should be stored at room temperature. (Chilled tubes could cause hemolysis.)

2. Fill tubes completely. If the tube is removed before the vacuum is exhausted, a rush of air can enter the tube and cause hemolysis.

3. Do not pull back too quickly on the plunger of a syringe, as this can cause hemolysis.

4. After completing a syringe draw, allow the vacuum in the tube to pull the blood into the tube. If blood is forced into the tube, hemolysis will result.

5. If it is difficult get the blood into the tube, i.e., slow fill, or difficult to find the location, reposition the needle and get a new tube.

6. Drawing blood with anything less than a 22 G could cause hemolysis. If it is necessary to use a smaller-sized gauge, use a smaller tube, i.e., a pediatric tube. A 21 G needle is probably the best choice to prevent hemolysis.

For information on vacutainer stoppers, colors, additives, and tube order refer to the Vacutainer Stopper Form, found later in this section.

BUTTERFLY METHOD

SUPPLIES

Butterfly needle	Syringe	Tape	Tubes	Cotton	Alcohol	Tourniquet
	Gloves	Adhesive bandage		Sharp's container		

WHEN TO USE THIS METHOD

1. This method is used many times in the same instances where a syringe would be used, i.e., in situations where patients have small or compromised veins or do not have visible or palpable veins in their arms but good veins in their hands.
2. This method is encouraged for patients who have a hard time holding still (e.g., children).

COMMON SITES

The antecubital veins in the arms, veins in the lower arm, and veins in the hands are common sites for this method of phlebotomy.

FACTS AND TROUBLESHOOTING TIPS

1. Make sure the vein is anchored firmly before attempting this procedure. (Veins used for this method tend to roll easier than those used for other methods.)
2. This procedure is much easier when two people perform the blood draw. One person inserts the needle and the other person pulls back the plunger, once blood enters the tubing.
3. Make sure the air has been expelled from the syringe before performing this procedure.
4. When using a needle smaller than 22 G, use pediatric tubes instead of standard-sized tubes. (This will help prevent hemolysis.)
5. Fill tubes that contain additive first.
6. Fill plain tubes last when performing this method.
7. Do not force blood into tubes. (This will cause hemolysis.)
8. Do not pull back on plunger too quickly. (This will cause hemolysis.)
9. Do not delay transferring the blood from the syringe into the tubes, or clotting may occur.
10. Apply gentle pressure for a minimum of two to three minutes following the blood draw and elevate the arm to minimize the risks of bruising or of acquiring a hematoma.
11. Follow all biohazard guidelines for the proper disposal of contaminated needles and supplies.

Any Modifications: _____

_____

_____

_____

_____

_____

Physician's Approval:_____

SYRINGE METHOD

SUPPLIES

Syringe	Needle	Tubes	Cotton	Tourniquet	Alcohol
	Adhesive bandage		Sharp's container	Gloves	

WHEN TO USE THIS METHOD

1. This is the method of choice in patients who have small veins.
2. This is the method of choice in patients whose veins collapse easily.
3. This is the preferred method in patients who have compromised veins, e.g., diabetics and elderly patients.

COMMON SITES

The antecubital veins, located in the arms, are the most common sites, however, veins in the lower arms and hands are sometimes used when employing the syringe method.

FACTS AND TROUBLESHOOTING TIPS

1. Fill tubes with additive first.
2. Plain tubes are filled last.
3. Do not pull back too quickly on the plunger. (This will cause hemolysis.)
4. Do not force blood into tubes. (This will cause hemolysis.)
5. Using one continuous motion helps reduce tissue damage.
6. Do not attempt to enter veins that are scarred, burned, bruised or close to areas where infection is present.
7. Avoid using veins where the patient complains of soreness or pain.
8. Remove the tourniquet before the needle to minimize internal and external bleeding at the puncture site.
9. Do not delay in transferring the blood from the syringe into the tubes, or clotting may occur.
10. Apply gentle pressure for a minimum of two to three minutes following a blood draw and elevate the arm to minimize the risks of bruising or of acquiring a hematoma.
11. Follow all biohazard guidelines for the proper disposal of contaminated needles and supplies.

Any Modifications: _____

_____

_____

_____

_____

_____

9

Physician's Approval:_____

CEPHALIC VEIN

MEDIAN CEPHALIC VEIN

SUPPLEMENTARY CEPHALIC VEIN

BASILIC VEIN

MEDIAN BASILIC VEIN

MEDIAN ANTEBRACHIAL VEIN

VACUTAINER METHOD

SUPPLIES

Plastic holder	Needle	Tubes	Cotton balls	Alcohol	Tourniquet
	Adhesive bandage		Sharp's container	Disposable gloves	

WHEN TO USE THIS METHOD

1. This is the preferred method for the majority of noncomplicated draws.
2. This is definitely the preferred method when multiple tubes are drawn.
3. This method should not be the method of choice when the patient has small veins or veins that easily collapse.

COMMON SITES

The antecubital veins, located in the arm. The median cephalic vein is the most common site used for the majority of blood draws.

FACTS AND TROUBLESHOOTING TIPS

1. Fill plain tubes first.
2. Fill tubes with additive last. If blue top tube is the only tube that is being drawn, a 5 ml discard tube should be drawn first to eliminate the possibility of thromboplastin contamination from the venipuncture site.
3. Do not attempt to enter veins that are scarred, burned, bruised or close to areas where infection is present. If patient already complains of soreness or pain in a certain area, avoid that area as well.
4. If the vein starts to swell while the needle is being inserted into the patient's arm, remove the tourniquet and withdraw the needle immediately. Apply pressure for several minutes following the stick. Choose a new site if there was not enough blood on the first draw.
5. Do not allow the tourniquet to stay on for more than one to two minutes. Remove the tourniquet while the first tube is filling, whenever possible.
6. If the vacuum tube is removed before the vacuum is exhausted, a rush of air can enter the tube and cause hemolysis.
7. Invert vacuum tube immediately to prevent hemolysis.
8. If the vacuum tube stops filling, readjust the needle. If the blood still does not flow into the tube, withdraw the old tube and insert a new tube.
9. Vacuum tubes should be stored at room temperature. (Chilled tubes may result in hemolysis.)
10. Try not to use any needles that are below 22 G, because of the danger of hemolysis.
11. To prevent the risk of bruising, have the patient apply pressure for a minimum of two to three minutes following the blood draw and elevate the arm.
12. Follow all biohazard guidelines for the disposal of contaminated needles and supplies.
13. If unsuccessful after two blood draws on the same person, alert the physician before reattempting.

Any Modifications: _____

_____

_____

_____

_____

_____

Physician's Approval:_____

TEST KIT GUIDELINES

Chemistry test kits vary from one kit to another. Before performing any lab tests, check with the physician for a current listing of waivered, moderate, and high complexity tests. The following is a list of general information regarding most test kits.

1. Read instruction thoroughly for each test kit.

2. Store the kit at the temperature listed in the instructions. (Some kits have to be room temperature, while other kits must be refrigerated.)

3. Check the expiration date before using the kit.

4. Always use reagents that were packaged with the kit. (Never use reagents that come from a different kit.)

5. Run controls as often as the directions instruct.

6. Be sure to follow instructions precisely. (Timing is very important with most test kits.)

7. Record test results in lab log. (This will help comply with the latest lab legislation.)

   Record the following information:

   a. name of patient

   b. lot # of test

   c. expiration date

   d. result of test

   e. name of physician who ordered test

   f. name of person who performed test

   g. control results (when applicable)

8. Record results on progress note (when applicable).

9. When in doubt, check with the physician. (Test may need to be redone.)

Section 12 contains a blank Test Kit Log for the assistant's convenience.

9

VACUTAINER STOPPER

STOPPER	SPECIMEN USAGE	ADDITIVE/ANTICOAGULANT
Red	Serological, blood chemistries, AIDS testing, viral studies, and blood typing	None; allow blood to clot for at least 30 minutes before spinning.
Red/Gray	Same as plain red (may be some exceptions; check lab reference manual to be certain)	Gel substance in bottom tube; also has clot activator on the interior walls of the tube. (Tubes should be inverted; allow blood to clot for a minimum of 30 minutes.)
Lavender	Most hematological procedures (CBC, sed rates, and platelet counts)	Liquid EDTA; the tube should be completely filled. Tube needs to be inverted.
Light Blue	Most coagulation studies, i.e., PT, PTT	Sodium citrate. Fill tube completely. This should never be the first tube drawn. (Draw a discard tube, if single tube.)
Green	Endocrine studies, blood gases, etc.	Sodium or ammonium heparin Fill tube completely. Tube needs to be inverted.
Gray	Blood glucose and alcohol levels	Sodium fluoride and potassium oxalate. Fill tube completely. Tube needs to be inverted.
Black	Westergren sed rate, i.e., malignancy, infectious disease, monitoring inflammatory disease	Sodium oxalate. Fill tube completely. Tube needs to be inverted.
Yellow	Blood cultures (check to see if there is any bacteria in the blood); some labs will have the assistant wipe off the stoppers with Betadine, as well as wipe the patient's arm, before performing the procedure.	Sodium polyanethanol-sulfonate (Do not contaminate this tube.) Fill tube completely and invert.

(continued on following page)

VACUTAINER STOPPER *(continued from previous page)*

Tube Order

The order in which tubes are filled is dictated by the method used and whether or not there is an additive.

Vacutainer Method:
1. Fill plain tubes before filling tubes with additive.
2. When a blood culture is ordered, always draw that tube first, then plain top tubes, and finally tubes that contain additive.
3. Coagulation studies such as PTs or PTTs should never be drawn first. If this test is ordered singly, draw off a small tube of blood first, then discard it.

EXAMPLE: (VACUTAINER ORDER)

1. Serum/clot/SST (red, red/black)
2. Na Citrate (blue, black)
3. Na Heparin (green)
4. Na Fluoride (gray)
5. EDTA (lavender)

Syringe and Butterfly Method:
1. Fill tubes with additive first. (This will help keep the blood from clotting.)
2. Fill PT and PTT tubes first, since the last part of the blood to come into the syringe will be the first blood that goes into the tube.
3. Never force blood into the tubes. (This will cause hemolysis.)

Number of Inversions:
1. This will vary depending on the lab. (Eight inversions appear to be average for most tubes.)
2. Check the lab reference manual for specifics.

Check the reference manual to see how blood is to be stored. (Some specimens must remain at room temperature, while other specimens must be frozen or refrigerated.) **Disclaimer: The above information is for illustrative purposes only. The medical assistant student should always double check the lab reference manual before performing any test.**

9

CHEMICAL URINALYSIS

EQUIPMENT

Gloves Chemical test strip Urine specimen

CONDITIONS THAT MAY CAUSE ABNORMAL TEST STRIP RESULTS

HEMOGLOBIN	BLOOD	UROBILINOGEN	BILIRUBIN	KETONES
Kidney dysfunctions, RBC hemolysis, blood transfusions that are incompatible, exposure to cold, and overexertion.	Kidney disease, trauma, infection, stones, tumors, and other urinary disorders, blood dyscrasias, some vitamin deficiencies, and vaginal contaminants.	Liver disease or trauma, hemolytic disease, and certain types of anemia.	Certain liver dysfunctions, biliary dysfunction, gallstones, and obstructive jaundice.	Starvation, vomiting and diarrhea, vigorous exercise, diabetic ketosis, toxemia, severe dieting, and acute fever.

GLUCOSE	PROTEIN	URINE pH	NITRITE	LEUKOCYTES
Renal tubular diseases and disorders, myocardial infarctions, sudden pain, diabetes mellitus, Cushing's syndrome, hyperthyroidism, and steroid therapy.	Renal diseases and disorders, CHF, preeclampsia, gout, hypokalemia, ingestion of various foods and drugs, and severe febrile infections.	Will be increased during bacterial infections of the kidney, alkalosis, and alkalizing drug use. Will be decreased with diarrhea, dehydration, malabsorption, starvation, certain diets, pulmonary emphysema, and acidifying drug use.	Will be positive during UTIs, kidney infections, urolithiasis, tumors, and prostatitis.	Will be positive during renal and urinary infections and various renal disorders.

FACTS AND TROUBLESHOOTING TIPS

1. Always check the expiration date before using test strips.

2. Tip urine container just slightly on its side and insert test strip so it is parallel with urine. (This is to keep test pads from running onto each other.)

3. Compare the test strip colors carefully with the chart. (Timing is critical.) Inaccurate results are oftentimes produced by not carefully timing each test.

4. Controls should be run as often as directed by the manufacturer.

5. Results should be carefully documented.

6. Test strip results should be logged in a special log book or notebook, in case any problems develop later on with those particular test strips. (Be sure to include a lot number with the results.)

(continued on following page)

CHEMICAL URINALYSIS *(continued from previous page)*

Any Modifications:

_____

_____

_____

_____

_____

Physician's Approval: _____

Courtesy of Miles Inc., Diagnostic Division

9

SECTION

10

LABORATORY TESTS AND VALUES

Introduction

The following section lists laboratory values for common chemistry and hematology tests. It also lists the clinical significance of each test. The normals that appear on the charts that follow were taken from a local reference laboratory. It is important to note that laboratory ranges vary from laboratory to laboratory, thus the assistant, when in doubt, should always check with the lab that is performing the test.

COMMON CHEMISTRY AND SEROLOGICAL TESTS

Test Name	Abbreviation	Range	Clinical Significance
Albumin	ALB	Adult 3.0-5.0 gm/dl Geriatric 3.5-4.5 gm/dl	Liver, kidney and nutritional status
Alkaline Phosphatase	ALP	Adult 30-130 U/L Children/Teens 75-450 U/L	Hepatobiliary disease and bone disease
Amylase		20-110 U/L	Pancreatitis and salivary gland disorders
Bilirubin Total	T Bil, TBili, Bili	0.3-1.3 mg/dl	Liver disease and hemolytic anemia
Bilirubin (Indirect)	IBili, IBili	0.00-1.20 mg/dl	
Bilirubin (Direct)	DBili, DBili	0.0-3.0	
Blood, Urea, Nitrogen	BUN	7-26 mg/dl	Kidney dysfunction, dehydration, GI bleeding
Calcium	Ca	8.5-10.5 mg/dl	Parathyroid disorders
Cancer Testing			
Carcinoembryonic Antigen	CEA	< 5.0 ng/ml smoker < 3.0 ng/ml nonsmoker	Various types of cancer
Prolactin Levels		0.0-25.0 ng/dl	Detection of prolactin-secreting tumors
Prostatic Specific Antigen	PSA	< 4.0 ng/ml	Prostate cancer and other prostate disorders
Lipids			
Cholesterol (Total)	CH., Chol	< 200 mg/dl	Coronary heart disease
High-Density Lipoprotein (good)	HDL	Female > 45 mg/dl Male > 36 mg/dl	Coronary heart disease
Low-Density Lipoprotein (bad)	LDL	< 130 mg/dl	Coronary heart disease
Triglycerides	Trig	30-150 mg/dl	Coronary heart disease, certain liver conditions, and pancreatitis
Creatinine	creat	0.7-1.5 mg/dl	Renal function

10

(continued on following page)

COMMON CHEMISTRY AND SEROLOGICAL TESTS *(continued from previous page)*

Test Name	Abbreviation	Range	Clinical Significance
Electrolytes	Elect, Lytes		
Sodium	Na	136-145 mEq/L	Diabetes insipidus, Addison's disease, diarrhea, and dehydration
Potassium	K+	3.5-5.0 mEq/L	Diuretic therapy, diarrhea, starvation, liver disease, etc.
Chloride	Cl⁻	101-111 mEq/L	Renal disease, diabetic acidosis, congestive heart failure, dehydration, anemia, severe diarrhea, and vomiting
Carbon Dioxide	CO	24-30 mEq/L	Electrolyte balance and respiratory disorders
Gamma Glutamyl Transpepetidase	GTP, GGT, GGTP	Male, 9-70 U/L Female, 5-45 U/L	Pancreatitis and liver disorders
Globulin	glob	1.5-3.5 g/dl	Rheumatoid arthritis, Hodgkin's disease, and chronic infections
Glucose	Gluc, Glu		
Fasting Blood Sugar	FBS	70-125 mg/dl	Diabetes; some liver and thyroid disorders
Random Blood Sugar	RBS	< 150 mg/dl	
Two-Hour Post Prandial Blood Sugar	2-hr PPBS	< 140 mg/dl	Diabetes
Glucose Tolerance Test	GTT	Fasting 70-125 mg/dl 30 minutes 150-160 mg/dl 1 hour 160-170 mg/dl 2 hours < 120 mg/dl 3 hours 70-125 mg/dl	Diabetes
Lactic Dehydrogenase	LDH, LD	Adults 100-225 U/L Children/ 150/350 U/L Teens	Pulmonary infarction, myocardial infarction, liver disease, muscular dystrophy, and pernicious anemia

(continued on following page)

COMMON CHEMISTRY AND SEROLOGICAL TESTS *(continued from previous page)*

Test Name	Abbreviation	Range	Clinical Significance
Magnesium	Mag, Mg	1.4-2.0 mEq/L	Malnutrition, diarrhea, alcoholism, pancreatitis, and prolonged gastric drainage
Phosphorus	P	30-45 mg/dl	Parathroid, renal, and diabetic disorders
Protein (Total)	TP, TPRO	Adult 6.5-8.0 gm/dl Child 3.0-6.0 gm/dl Geriatric 6.1-7.9 gm/dl	Dehydration, multiple myeloma, nephrotic syndrome, severe burns, and extensive bleeding
Serum Glutamic-Oxaloacetic Transaminase	SGOT, AST	0-41 U/L	Myocardial infarction, muscular dystrophy, infectious mononucleosis, and various liver disorders
Serum Glutamic-Pyruvic Transaminase	SGPT, ALT	1-45 U/L	Liver disorders, myocardial infarction, and muscular dystrophy
Thyroid-Stimulating Hormone	TSH	0.3-4.5 mIU/dl	Thyroid and certain pituitary disorders
Thyroxine	T_3	4.5-13.0 ug/dl	Thyroid disorders
Triiodothyronine	T_4	Total: 60-180 mg/ml Uptake 27-42 % or 0.9-2.0 ng/ml	Thyroid disorders
Triglyceride	Trig	30-150 mg/dl	Coronary heart disease, certain liver conditions, and pancreatitis
Uric Acid	UA	Male 3.4-7.5 mg/dl Female 2.4-6.5 mg/dl Child 2.0-6.0 mg/dl	Renal failure, gout, leukemia, eclampsia, and lymphomas

10

ROUTINE HEMATOLOGY TESTS

TEST	DESCRIPTION		RANGES
Hematocrit (Hct)	Measures the packed red blood cell volume	Men	38-51%
		Women	36-47%
		Neonates	44-70%
Hemoglobin (Hgb)	Measures the iron concentration found on the RBCS	Men	13.5-17.0 g/dl
		Women	12.0-16.0 g/dl
		Neonates	15.0-24.0 g/dl
RBC Count	Measures the total # of RBCs /cumm	Men	4.4-6.0 mill/mm3
		Women	4.0-5.5 mill/mm3
		Neonates	4.0-6.6 mill/mm3
WBC Count	Measures the total # of WBCs/cumm	Male and Female	4,000-10,000
		Neonates	9,000-25,000
MCV	Measures the average volume of RBCs per liter	Male and Female	78-96%
		Neonates	100-115%
MCH	Is a measure of the average hemoglobin content on the RBC	Male and Female	27-34 PG
		Neonates	33-39 PG
MCHC	A measure of the average hemoglobin content per unit volume of RBCs		32-36%
Differential	Increased in bacterial and parasitic infections and liver disease	Segs	45-75%
Neutrophil	Decreased in viral infections, hormone diseases, and chemotherapy	Bands	0-5 %

(continued on following page)

ROUTINE HEMATOLOGY TESTS *(continued from previous page)*

TEST	DESCRIPTION	RANGES
Lymphocyte	Increased in viral infections, hyperthyroidism, carcinoma, hematopoetic disorders, and Addison's disease; decreased in HIV infection, leukemia, cardiac failure, Cushing's disease, and Hodgkin's disease	15-40%
Monocytes	Increased in certain bacterial infections Decreased in chemotherapy	0-10%
Eosinophils	Increased in allergic reactions, parasitic infections, lung and bone cancer, and Addison's disease Decreased in infectious mononucleosis, CHF, hypersplenism, and aplastic anemia	0-6%
Basophil	Increased in leukemia, hemolytic anemia, and chronic inflammation	0-2%
Erythrosedimentation Rate (ESR)	Measures how fast the RBCs fall in a given amount of time. (Helps in the detection and monitoring of disease, especially occult diseases, infection, and rheumatoid arthritis.)	Westergren's method, Males 0-20 mm/h; Females 0-30 mm/h
Prothrombin Time (PT)	Checks for coagulation disorders and also helps monitor patients who are on anticoagulation therapy, i.e., Coumadin therapy.	11-16 seconds
Platelet Count	Helps evaluate various bleeding disorders	150,000-440,000/cumm

10

SECTION

11

DIAGNOSTIC IMAGING

Introduction

This section will benefit those who are not familiar with Xray, ultrasound, CT, and MRI examinations. A list of terms and definitions, common patient preparations, and descriptions of these exams will aid the assistant in providing valuable advice to patients. This section also includes standard information that needs to be obtained before scheduling exams. Because of the differences in health insurance, preauthorization of procedures may be necessary. (Check with the patient before scheduling.) For procedures that may not be covered by the patient's health insurance, a waiver must be obtained from the patient, with his or her signature, stating that any fee not covered by the insurance company will be paid by the patient.

Since the examination/preparation instructions listed are general (and often change), it is wise to check with the facility for specific instructions.

INFORMATION NEEDED WHEN ORDERING XRAYS

1. Name of Xray to be ordered and who ordered it.
2. Probable diagnosis or what the doctor is looking for.
3. What symptoms or signs lead the physician to his or her probable diagnosis.
4. Patient's telephone number and address.
5. Name and age of patient or date of birth.
6. Patient's social security number and insurance information.

Many insurance companies precertify specific Xrays. Check with the insurance company's guidelines before sending a patient for Xrays.

POSITIONING TERMS AND ABBREVIATIONS

1. Supine position: Patient is placed on his or her back with the face pointing upward.
2. Prone position: Patient is placed with the face pointed downward and to the side.
3. Oblique: Patient is positioned in a semilateral position or at an angle.
4. Lateral: The beam goes from one side of the body to the other.
5. Right Lateral (RL): The right side of the body is positioned next to the film and the Xray tube is placed toward the left side of the body so the rays will travel from the left side of the body to the right side.
6. Left Lateral (LL): The left side of the body is positioned next to the film and the Xray tube is placed toward the right side of the body so the rays will travel from the right side of the body to the left side.
7. Posteroanterior view (PA): The Xray tube is placed toward the posterior portion of the body with the film toward the anterior aspect of the body.
8. Anteroposterior view (AP): The Xray tube is placed toward the anterior portion of the body with the film toward the posterior aspect of the body.

Disclaimer: All patients having Xrays should be provided with lead shielding, when permitted, particularly in the gonadal region.

All patients should have consent forms explained and signed, when indicated.

ROUTINE FLAT FILMS

PREPARATIONS

IMPORTANT NOTE: The following preps list only general information; always double check with the Xray facility before providing specific instructions to the patient. (Procedures vary from one facility to another.)

Prep A: Ten-day rule for females twelve and above: (Day 1 of menses to Day 10 of menses is considered a safe time to take Xrays.) Inquire about birth control. If the patient is past Day 10 of cycle, a urine pregnancy test should be performed prior to taking the Xray. (If the test is positive, Xrays should not be taken.)

Prep B: Remove false teeth, necklaces, and earrings prior to taking the Xray.

Prep C: Remove necklaces and earrings prior to taking the Xray.

Prep D: Do not apply any deodorants, lotions, or powders to breasts or underarms prior to Xray.

Prep E: Nothing by mouth after midnight.

Prep F: Fluids only the day before Xray; take laxatives as directed.

Prep G: Laxative or cathartic given the night before or the morning of the exam.

Prep H: Do not take vitamins that contain iodine four weeks prior to testing, per physician's orders. Patient will be given one to two capsules containing a radioactive iodine prior to testing.

Prep I: Ask if the patient is allergic to iodine.

Viewing sections will vary from one facility to another

TYPE	DESCRIPTION	PREP
Cervical spine	Various views are taken on C1-T1	A
Thoracic spine	Various views are taken on T1-T12	A
Lumbar spine	AP and lateral views are taken on T12-L1 and a lateral spot of L-5 and S-1 is also taken.	A
Extremities	Anterior, posterior, and oblique views are taken on the extremities involved.	A
KUB (flat abdomen)	Views allow visualization of the kidneys, ureters, and bladder	A
Sinus films	Various views allow visualization of the sinuses	A, B
Chest Xray	Posterior and left lateral views are taken of the chest.	A, C

(continued on following page)

ROUTINE FLAT FILMS *(continued from previous page)*

TYPE	DESCRIPTION	PREP
Mammogram	Xray views are taken of the breast from two angles.	A, D
Barium swallow	Xray of the esophagus only. May be ordered with upper GI series.	A, E
Upper GI series	Xray of the stomach and small intestine. May be ordered with barium swallow and/or small bowel follow-through.	A, E
Barium enema	Xray of the large colon only. May be ordered with air contrast, which means gas is inserted into the colon to extend it.	A, E, F
IVP	Intravenous Pyelogram. Xray of the kidneys, ureters, and bladder. Intravenous contrast is used, i.e., iodine.	A, E, G, I
Gallbladder series	Xray of gallbladder after oral ingestion of radiopaque, iodinated dye in the form of a pill. (This test is slowly being phased out; refer to gallbladder ultrasound.)	A, E, H, I
Thyroid uptake or thyroid scan	Evaluates overall function of the thyroid and detects any abnormalities.	A, H, I

ULTRASOUND

Ultrasound uses ultrasonic waves to produce an image of an organ or tissue for diagnostic examination.

PREPARATIONS

Prep A: Nothing by mouth after midnight.

Prep B: No carbonated beverages the day before the procedure.

Prep C: Low-fat meal the night before the test.

Prep D: One to two quarts of water two hours before the exam. Do not urinate before the ultrasound is performed.

TYPE	DESCRIPTION	PREP
Abdominal	Can view liver, gallbladder, spleen, or pancreas	A, B, C
Renal Ultrasound	Able to view entire kidney	A, B
Pelvic Ultrasound	Able to view bladder, ureters, ovaries, fallopian tubes, and uterus	B, D
Echocardiogram	Used to evaluate the structure and function of the heart	None
Thyroid Ultrasound	Distinguishes cystic from solid thyroid nodules	None

COMPUTERIZED TOMOGRAPHY (CT SCAN)

Computer-constructed imaging technique allows visualization of bone tissue, soft tissue, and internal organs.

PREPARATIONS

Prep A: Nothing by mouth four hours before test.

Prep B: Ten-day rule for female patients twelve and above. Day 1-10 of menstrual cycle is considered a safe time to take Xrays. If the patient's last menstrual period is past the 10-day mark, a urine pregnancy test should be performed prior to Xraying the patient. If test is positive, *do not perform the test.*

Prep C: Patient is given an oral contrast, either the night before or several hours before the Xray is performed; or IV dye may be administered.

Prep D: Ask if patient is allergic to seafood (iodine).

TYPE

TYPE	PREP
Brain CT	A, B, C, D
Body CT	A, B
Chest CT	A, B, C, D
Abdomen/Pelvic CT	A, B, C, D

MAGNETIC RESONANCE IMAGING (MRI)

No radiation; uses a strong magnet and radiowaves that cannot be felt. MRIs produce computerized images that can be displayed immediately and stored on file and/or magnetic tape. MRIs can be done on any area of the body.

PREPARATIONS

Patient needs to remove anything that may be affected by a magnet, such as watches, jewelry, credit cards, keys, bobby pins, and coins. Patients who have aneurism clips, pacemakers, surgical clips, or a prosthesis *cannot* have MRIs.

SECTION

12

BLANK FORMS

ABC Insurance Company
Pre-Certification Form

Pre-Certification/
Authorization #: _____   Date of Authorization: _____

Patient's Name:_____   Date of Birth: _____

Patient's ID #: _____   Primary Care Physician: _____

Employer: _____

Diagnosis:_____   Diagnosis Code: _____

Procedure:_____   Procedure Code: _____

Name of facility/physician the patient is being referred to:

_____

_____

Provider Relation's Representative:_____

Plan Information Form

Plan Representative: _____

Phone #: _____

Procedures That Require Pre-Certification:

_____	_____
_____	_____
_____	_____
_____	_____
_____	_____
_____	_____
_____	_____
_____	_____
_____	_____
_____	_____
_____	_____

Participating Providers

Labs: _____   Phone: _____
      _____   Phone: _____

Xray: _____   Phone: _____
      _____   Phone: _____

Pharmacies: _____   Phone: _____
      _____   Phone: _____

Hospitals: _____   Phone: _____
      _____   Phone: _____
      _____   Phone: _____
      _____   Phone: _____

Specialists: _____   Phone: _____
      _____   Phone: _____
      _____   Phone: _____
      _____   Phone: _____
      _____   Phone: _____

GENERAL COMPLAINT FORM

COLUMN 1	COLUMN 2	COLUMN 3
QUESTIONS	POSSIBLE PROCEDURES	TELEPHONE TRIAGE

Any Modifications:

Physician's Approval: _____

PEDIATRIC ROUTINE PROCEDURES FORM

Age	HC	WT	HT	PP	LAB TESTS	ROUTINE PROCEDURES
NB						
1 mo						
2 mo						
3 mo						
4 mo						
6 mo						
9 mo						
12 mo						
15 mo						
18 mo						
4-6 yrs						
11-12 yrs						
14-16 yrs						

Any Modifications:

Physician's Approval: _____

GENERAL PEDIATRIC ASSESSMENT FORM

Call EMS	Should Be Seen in Office ASAP	(Same Day—24 Hours)	(Within the Week)

(continued on following page)

GENERAL PEDIATRIC ASSESSMENT FORM *(continued from previous page)*

Call EMS	Should Be Seen in Office ASAP	(Same Day—24 Hours)	(Within the Week)

Any Modifications:

Physician's Approval: _____

OVER-THE-COUNTER ADULT CHART

Before using this chart, read the OTC Medication Instruction Sheet.

ADULT COUGH SYRUPS

BRAND NAME	RECOMMENDED DOSAGE
1.	
2.	
3.	

ADULT PAIN RELIEVERS AND ANTIPYRETICS

BRAND NAME	RECOMMENDED DOSAGE
1.	
2.	
3.	

ADULT ANTIHISTAMINE FORMULAS

BRAND NAME	RECOMMENDED DOSAGE
1.	
2.	
3.	

ADULT COLD FORMULAS

BRAND NAME	RECOMMENDED DOSAGE
1.	
2.	
3.	

(continued on following page)

12

OVER-THE-COUNTER ADULT CHART *(continued from previous page)*

ADULT ANTACIDS

BRAND NAME	RECOMMENDED DOSAGE
1.	
2.	
3.	

ADULT VAGINAL CREAMS

BRAND NAME	RECOMMENDED DOSAGE
1.	
2.	
3.	

ADULT TOPICAL CREAMS

1. POISON IVY	
2. LACERATIONS	
3. BURNS	

Physician's Approval: _____

OVER-THE-COUNTER PEDIATRIC CHART

Before using this chart, read the OTC Medication Instruction Sheet.

PEDIATRIC COUGH SYRUPS

BRAND NAME	RECOMMENDED DOSAGE
1.	
2.	
3.	

PEDIATRIC PAIN RELIEVERS AND ANTIPYRETICS

BRAND NAME	RECOMMENDED DOSAGE
1.	
2.	
3.	

PEDIATRIC ANTIHISTAMINE FORMULAS

BRAND NAME	RECOMMENDED DOSAGE
1.	
2.	
3.	

PEDIATRIC COLD FORMULAS

BRAND NAME	RECOMMENDED DOSAGE
1.	
2.	
3.	

(continued on following page)

12

OVER-THE-COUNTER PEDIATRIC CHART *(continued from previous page)*

PEDIATRIC ANTACIDS

BRAND NAME	RECOMMENDED DOSAGE
1.	
2.	
3.	

PEDIATRIC TOPICAL CREAMS

1. POISON IVY	
2. BURNS	
3. LACERATIONS	
4. DIAPER RASH	

Physician's Approval: _____

TEST KIT LOG

Date	Lot #	Expiration Date	Patient's Name	Physician's Initials	Test Results	Performer's Initials

References

American Druggist, July 1994, 33-41.

Baldwin-Brown, J. (1995). The obstetric history. *PMA, Professional Medical Assistant,* September/October.

Bonewit-West, K. (1995). *Clinical procedures for medical assistants* (4th ed.). Philadelphia, PA: W. B. Saunders.

Colbert, B. J., Ankney, J., Wilson, J., & Havrilla, J. (1997). *An integrated approach to health sciences: Anatomy and physiology, math, physics, and chemistry.* Albany, NY: Delmar Publishers.

Diagnostic tests handbook. (1993). Springhouse, PA: Springhouse Corporation.

Fordney, M.T., and Follis, J. J. (1993). *Administrative medical assisting* (3rd ed.) Albany, NY: Delmar Publishers.

Guidelines for health supervision. (1985). Elkgrove Village, IL: American Academy of Pediatrics.

Katz, H. P. (1990). *Telephone medicine: Triage and training—A handbook for primary care health professionals.* Philadelphia, PA: F. A. Davis.

Keir, L., Wise, B. A., and Krebs, C. (1993). *Medical assisting: Administrative and clinical competencies* (3rd ed.) Albany, NY: Delmar Publishers.

Lane, K. (1992). *Medications: A guide for the health professions.* Philadelphia, PA: F. A. Davis.

Merck manual. (1992). West Point, PA: Merck Co. Inc.

Mosby's medical, nursing, & allied health dictionary (4th ed.) (1994). St. Louis, MO: Mosby Year Book, Inc.

1994 Red Book, Elkgrove Village, IL: American Academy of Pediatrics. 1994.

Physician's Office Laboratory Procedure Manual. (1992). NCCLS Document POL2-T2. 12(7).

Rice, J. (1994). *Principles of pharmacology for medical assisting.* (2nd ed.). Albany, NY: Delmar Publishers.

Spratto, G. R., & Woods, A. L. (1996). *Delmar's drug guide for nurses* 1996. Albany, NY: Delmar Publishers.

The Merck manual. (16th ed.) (1992). Rahway, NJ: Merck Research Laboratories.

Top 200 drugs of 1995. *Pharmacy Times,* April 1996, 29–36.

Tuttle-Yoder, J. A., & Fraser-Nobbe, S. A. (1996). *STAT medical office emergency manual.* Albany, NY: Delmar Publishers.

Wedding, M. E., & Toenjes, S. A. (1992). *Medical laboratory procedures.* Philadelphia, PA: F. A. Davis.

COMMON ABBREVIATIONS *(continued from inside front cover)*

M

M mix; minimum, married; medication
MA mental age
mcg microgram; one millionth gram
meds medication
mEq/L milliequivalent (per liter)
mg milligram; one thousandth gram
MH medical, marital, menstrual history
mmHg millimeter of mercury
ml milliliter
mm millimeter
MM mucous membrane
MMR measles, mumps, rubella
mo month
mono mononucleosis
MS multiple sclerosis

N

N negative
NA not applicable
NaCl sodium chloride
NAD no appreciable disease
NB newborn
NC no change
neg negative
net internet
NG nasogastric
NKA no known allergies
NKDA no known drug allergies
NL normal limits
N/O no complaints
no show did not show up
noc night
nox (at) night
NPC nasopharyngeal culture
NPN non-protein nitrogen
NSR normal sinus rhythm
NTG nitroglycerin
N/V nausea and vomiting
NYD not yet diagnosed

O

OB obstetrics
OC office call; oral contraceptive
occ occasional
OD right eye
ofc office
OP operation; operative; outpatient

OPD outpatient department
OR operating room
orig original
os mouth
OS left eye
OS office surgery
OTC over-the-counter
OU both eyes (each eye)
OV office visit
oz ounce

P

p after
P pulse; primary, pupil
P&A percussion and auscultation
PA posterior artery; posteroanterior
PAP Papanicolaou
PARA 1 for the first time pregnant
PAT pre-admission testing
Path pathology
PBI protein-bound iodine
pc after meals
PC personal computer; present complaint
pcb please call back
PCN penicillin
PCV packed cell volume
PD permanent disability
pdr powder
PE physical examination
ped pediatric
perf performed
PERRLA pupils equal, round, react to light and accommodation
pH hydrogen-ion concentration
PH past history
Ph ex physical examination
PI present illness
PID pelvic inflammatory disease
PKU phenylketonuria
PLBO placebo
pls please
PM afternoon
PND postnasal drip
po by mouth, orally
PO postoperative
POL physician's office laboratory
POMR problem-oriented medical record

P Op postoperative
powd powder
PP postprandial
PPBS postprandial blood sugar
PPE personal protective equipment
preop preoperative
prep prepare; preparation
PRN as needed
Pro time prothrombin time
prog prognosis
P&S permanent and stationary
Psych psychiatry
pt patient; pint
PT physical therapy
PTR patient to return
pulv powder
PVC premature ventricular contraction
pwd powder
PX physical examination

Q

q every
QA quality assurance; qualitative analysis
QC quality control
qd every day
qh every hour
qns quantity not sufficient
qod every other day
qs quantity sufficient
qt quart

R

R respiration, right
Ra radium
RBC red blood cell; red blood count
RBS random blood sugar
re: regarding
REC recommend
re-ch re-check
re-exam re-examination
reg regular
REM rapid eye movement
rep let it be repeated
ret return
rev review
RHD rheumatic heart disease
RLQ right lower quadrant
R/O rule out